Melanoma - Standard of Care, Challenges, and Updates in Clinical Research

Edited by Sonia Maciá and Eduardo Castañón

Published in London, United Kingdom

Melanoma - Standard of Care, Challenges, and Updates in Clinical Research
http://dx.doi.org/10.5772/intechopen.100843
Edited by Sonia Maciá and Eduardo Castañón

Contributors
Hiu Kwan Carolyn Tang, Joon Wee Ho, Tatjana Zablocka, Sergejs Isajevs, Gerardo Cazzato, Anna Colagrande, Lucia Lospalluti, Giuseppe Ingravallo, Caterina Foti, Leonardo Resta, Eliano Cascardi, Miriam Dellino, Eugenio Maiorano, Saverio Capodiferro, Kasimu Umar Adoke, Dan-Corneliu Jinga, Maria-Ruxandra Jinga, Darina Lysková, Paulína Plesníková, Viera Horvathova Kajabova, Lucia Demkova, Božena Smolková, Jela Valášková, Sonia Maciá, Álvaro Sánchez Arráez, Eduardo Castañón, Ali Khani Jeihooni, Pooyan Afzali Harsini, Gholamreza Imani, Saeed Hamzehie, Monal Depani, James F. Thornton

First published in London, United Kingdom, 2023 by IntechOpen
IntechOpen is the global imprint of INTECHOPEN LIMITED, registered in England and Wales, registration number: 11086078, 5 Princes Gate Court, London, SW7 2QJ, United Kingdom

British Library Cataloguing-in-Publication Data
A catalogue record for this book is available from the British Library

Additional hard and PDF copies can be obtained from orders@intechopen.com

Melanoma - Standard of Care, Challenges, and Updates in Clinical Research
Edited by Sonia Maciá and Eduardo Castañón
p. cm.
Print ISBN 978-1-80356-398-5
Online ISBN 978-1-80356-399-2
eBook (PDF) ISBN 978-1-80356-400-5

Meet the editors

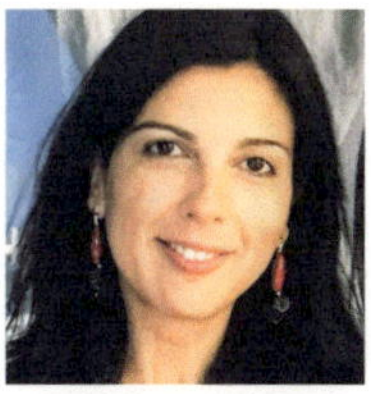

Sonia Maciá is an ESMO-certified medical oncologist. She obtained a master's degree in pharmacoeconomics from Universitat Pompeu Fabra Barcelona and a Ph.D. in lung cancer from the University Miguel Hernández. She has an Executive MBA from EAE/University of Barcelona. Dr. Maciá worked as a practicing medical oncologist for nine years and then decided to devote her career to clinical research. After working for different CROs, she joined Highlight Therapeutics to work on clinical development for intratumoral immunotherapies. Currently, Dr. Maciá is Executive Medical Director at LAVA Therapeutics, working on early development with several immunotherapies for solid and hematologic malignancies. Dr. Maciá has submitted more than 40 abstracts to international conferences, published more than 30 papers in peer-reviewed journals, and authored six book chapters.

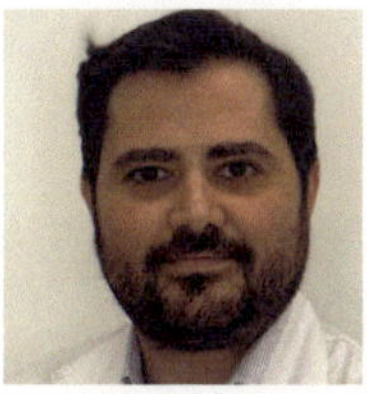

Eduardo Castañón, is an ESMO-certified medical oncologist. He obtained his Ph.D. in lung cancer at the University of Navarra, a master's degree in research methods from the Universidad Autónoma de Barcelona, a master's degree in molecular oncology from Universidad Rey Juan Carlos and a master's degree in big-data science from the University of Navarra. Following two years spent in the Early Phase I Trial Unit in Gustave Roussy (DITEP), supervised by Professor Jean Charles Soria, he is currently working in the Phase I trial Unit in Clínica Universidad de Navarra. Dr. Castañón is the author of more than 50 papers and several book chapters and has contributed over 50 abstracts to international conferences.

Contents

Preface

Melanoma is a severe type of skin cancer originating in cells called melanocytes. Despite being less prevalent than other skin tumors, melanoma is more deadly due to its tendency to migrate to other organs without rapid and early treatment.

This book presents the most relevant and up-to-date aspects of the epidemiology, diagnosis, biomarkers and treatment of melanoma, including specific sections on prognostic features and novel therapies, as well as particular clinical situations leading to a poor prognosis, such as brain metastases, or specific scenarios, such as uveal melanoma.

An accurate diagnosis is key and will determine both the prognosis and treatment landscape for each patient. The histopathological diagnosis of malignant melanoma remains the gold standard allowing the patient to access the entire diagnostic-therapeutic assistance process. Standard approaches are examined, as well as challenging situations which remain complex to diagnose. The various criteria used by dermatopathologists are also discussed.

As a systemic treatment, immunotherapy is part of the new therapeutic options that have significantly improved the prognosis of metastatic melanoma patients. The book reviews traditional immunotherapeutic approaches and focuses on immune checkpoint inhibitors such as anti-CTLA-4 inhibitors, anti-PD-1 inhibitors in monotherapy or in combination (dual immune blockade), presenting the key data that have achieved regulatory approval for current standard immunotherapies. Other systemic treatment options are also summarized, and a treatment algorithm based on American (NCCN) and European (ESMO) guidelines is provided, underlining the first, second and subsequent lines of treatment for both melanoma subtypes (BRAF wild type and mutated) and for particular cases, such as in-transit metastasis or brain metastasis. Special attention is given to treatment options for early and late disease progression (primary and acquired resistance after adjuvant therapy).

Beyond the standard approved treatments, recent advances in melanoma are also presented in this book. Systemic and local treatments undergoing clinical development, with their mechanisms of action, are included, together with preliminary or final results that have been presented, most of them in terms of response rate. Research has dramatically improved the prognosis in these patients, and we must all continue working in this direction to help our patients and further improve their responses and survival.

Thanks are due to the authors for their valuable contribution and commitment to providing a clear and succinct overview of these topics.

Dr. Sonia Maciá
LAVA Therapeutics,
Utrecht, The Netherlands

Dr. Eduardo Castañón
Clínica Universidad de Navarra,
Madrid, Spain

Section 1

Diagnosis and Clinical Characteristics

Chapter 1

Melanoma Epidemiology: Symptoms, Causes, and Preventions

Ali Khani Jeihooni, Pooyan Afzali Harsini, Gholamreza Imani and Saeed Hamzehie

Abstract

Melanoma arises from melanocyte cells. Melanoma spreads faster than basal cell carcinoma (BCC) and squamous cell carcinoma (SCC) if not diagnosed and treated early. Melanocyte tumors cause malignant melanoma. The preponderance of these cells is in the skin, gut, and eye. Melanoma is a rare kind of skin cancer, although it causes 75% of skin cancer deaths. Melanocytes create melanin, a dark pigment, in the skin. Despite years of lab and clinical research, early surgical removal of tiny cancers remains the most successful treatment. The deadliest skin cancer is melanoma. Skin melanocytes are involved. Melanocytes produce skin pigment melanin. Melanin protects skin against ultraviolet (UV) radiation. Skin cancer is the most common form in the United States. When diagnosed early, skin cancer can be treated with topical medications, office therapies, or outpatient surgery. Dermatologists treat skin disorders and conditions. Skin cancer causes less than 1% of cancer fatalities. Detection and treatment of melanoma in its early stages are typically curable. Once melanoma spreads further into the skin or other organs, it becomes incurable and potentially lethal. Early detection of melanoma in the United States is anticipated to result in a 5-year survival rate of roughly 99%.

Keywords: Cancer, skin cancer, cancer prevention, Melanoma, BCC, SCC

1. Introduction

Melanoma is a form of skin cancer that manifests itself when melanocytes, the cells responsible for giving the skin its brown or tanned appearance, begin to increase uncontrollably.

When cells in the body begin to develop uncontrolled, this is the beginning stage of cancer. Cancer can start in cells in virtually any part of the body, and once it does, it can quickly travel to other body parts [1].

Melanoma is one of the rarest forms of skin cancer, especially compared to other types. Melanoma, on the other hand, poses a greater threat since it has a greater potential to metastasize or spread to other areas of the body if it is not detected and treated in its early stages [2].

When usually healthy cells incur mutations and begin to increase uncontrollably, a mass known as a tumor forms. There are two different sorts of tumors: benign and malignant. Malignant tumors have the ability to metastasize or spread to other parts of the body. The term "benign" means that a tumor can develop but will not spread [3].

More than three million people in the United States are diagnosed with skin cancer each year, making it the most prevalent form of the disease. When detected at an early stage, skin cancer is typically amenable to treatment with topical medicines, treatments performed in the office by a dermatologist, or surgery performed on an outpatient basis. A physician who specializes in treating diseases and ailments that affect the skin is called a dermatologist. Because of this, skin cancer is responsible for fewer than 1% of the total deaths caused by cancer [4, 5].

A dermatologist, a surgical oncologist, a radiation oncologist, and a medical oncologist are typical members of the multidisciplinary teams that are required to address more advanced instances of skin cancer, which can occur under certain circumstances [6]. These physicians will consult with the patient to determine the most effective strategy for treating cancer and present their findings to the patient. When the operation to treat the cancer is too comprehensive to be conducted in an office environment, the surgical oncologist may suggest that the patient undergo surgery instead. This is one of the situations in which an operating room is required. At other times, the team will propose radiation therapy and/or other therapies using medication that is either taken orally or delivered intravenously as an alternative to or in combination with surgery [7].

2. Melanoma

Melanoma is a severe kind of skin cancer originating in cells called melanocytes [8]. Despite being less prevalent than basal cell carcinoma (BCC) and squamous cell carcinoma (SCC), melanoma is more deadly due to its tendency to migrate to other organs if not treated early rapidly. Melanoma is a tumor of melanocytes that is malignant [9]. These cells are primarily found in the skin, as well as in the intestine and the eye. Melanoma is one of the less prevalent forms of skin cancer, although it is responsible for most (75%) of skin cancer-related fatalities [10]. Melanocytes are generally present in the skin and are responsible for synthesizing melanin, a dark pigment. Despite many years of extensive laboratory and clinical research, early surgical removal of thin cancers continues to offer the best chance of cure. Melanoma is the most dangerous kind of skin cancer [11]. It begins in the melanocytes of the skin. Melanocytes are the cells responsible for producing melanin, which gives skin its color. Melanin protects the skin's deeper layers from the sun's ultraviolet (UV) radiation [12].

Melanocytes produce two different types of melanin: the black/brown pigment eumelanin and the red/yellow pigment pheomelanin. In contrast to the number of melanocytes, which is largely constant in all skin types, the ratio of eumelanin to pheomelanin in the skin influences skin color. People with darker skin have a lower risk of developing skin cancer, because the darker eumelanin serves as a better UV protection. In addition to providing less protection against UV light, pheomelanin synthesis also creates carcinogens [13].

It has been demonstrated that pheomelanin increases the amount of ultraviolet-A-induced reactive oxidative species (ROS) that cause DNA damage in response to UV exposure [14]. Melanoma risk has long been associated with skin, hair, and eye coloration: those with light skin that does not tan, blond or red hair, and light eyes have a significantly higher risk of developing the disease than the general population [15].

MC1R is partially responsible for regulating skin, hair, and eyes color. The amount of activity of the MC1R gene is controlled by polymorphisms. Reduced MC1R function caused by MC1R gene variations causes the development of mostly red/yellow pheomelanin pigment, fair skin that does not tan, and light eyes and hair. A fully functional MC1R stimulates eumelanin production. Due to greater exposure of the nuclei to UV radiation, individuals with less functioning MC1R variations accrue more mutations. Skin tumors may develop if mutations gather in the genome's susceptible areas [16].

Only 22.1 out of every 100,000 people in the United States are affected by melanoma, a malignant tumor that develops from melanocytes (cancer statistics from the Center for Disease Control and Prevention). Even though it only accounts for 4% of skin cancer incidences, it is a very fatal illness that causes 75% of skin cancer deaths. There are anticipated to be 96,480 new cases of melanoma detected in 2019 and 7230 fatalities in the United States alone (American Cancer Society). This overview will cover the major methods for diagnosing melanoma, patient prognosis, significant molecular flaws contributing to melanoma progression, and therapy options for melanoma [17].

Melanocytes are skin cells located in the epidermis [18]. They create the pigment melanin, which is responsible for the color of skin. Two types of melanin exist The pigments eumelanin and pheomelanin. Exposure to ultraviolet (UV) radiation from the sun or tanning beds causes skin damage that stimulates melanocytes to make more melanin. However, only the eumelanin pigment aims to protect the skin by darkening or tanning the skin. Melanoma develops when melanocytes incur mutations due to sunburn or tanning-induced DNA damage, leading to uncontrolled cell growth [19].

Early detection and treatment of melanoma is frequently curative. Once melanoma has migrated further into the skin or to other organs, it becomes more difficult to cure and potentially fatal. The expected 5-year survival rate for US patients diagnosed with melanoma early is approximately 99%.

In 2022, an estimated 7650 Americans (5080 males and 2570 women) would succumb of melanoma [20].

When people are exposed to sunshine, their melanocytes produce more melanin, causing their skin to tan. This also occurs while exposing to other ultraviolet radiation (such as in a tanning booth). If the skin is exposed to an excessive amount of ultraviolet radiation, the melanocytes may begin to grow abnormally and develop cancer. This disease is known as melanoma [19].

Approximately 60,000 new cases of invasive melanoma are detected annually in the United States, with males and Caucasians being affected more commonly. It is more prevalent among Caucasian communities living in sunny climates or in individuals who frequent tanning salons than in other ethnicities [21].

According to a WHO estimate, over 48,000 people die annually from melanoma. The treatment consists of tumor excision, adjuvant therapy, chemo- and immunotherapy, or radiation therapy [22].

When people are exposed to sunshine, their melanocytes produce more melanin, causing their skin to tan [19]. This also occurs when other forms of UV radiation are present (such as in a tanning booth). The melanocytes may begin to grow abnormally and develop cancer if the skin is exposed to an excessive amount of UV light. This condition is referred to as melanoma.

Each year, around 60,000 new instances of invasive melanoma are diagnosed in the United States, with males and Caucasians being disproportionately impacted [23]. It is more common among Caucasian cultures living in sunny climes or those who visit tanning salons than among other ethnic groups.

3. Diagnosis and prognosis of melanoma

Early melanoma classification was based on the origin of the tumor (existing nevus, acquired melanocytic lesion, and blemish-free skin); however, in the 1960s, a prominent dermatologist, Wallace Clark, proposed that melanoma should be classified based on its histological characteristics, thereby revolutionizing melanoma diagnosis.

To begin, he classified melanoma into three distinct subtypes based on their histological appearance: superficial spreading melanoma (SSM), lentigo maligna melanoma (LMM), and nodular melanoma (NM). Clark was the first to recognize that melanoma is a heterogeneous illness, showing that the variations behave differently and have distinct prognosticates and distinct treatments. Since then, several new variants have been identified, including acral lentiginous melanoma, mucosal melanoma, desmoplastic melanoma, and nevoid melanoma. On the second tier, we have noses and the fact that not all melanomas require the same treatment [24].

Clark also suggested a method for assessing melanoma in 1966 that takes into account the depth to which melanoma cells have penetrated the dermis and subcutaneous fat. Clark identified histologically distinguishable anatomic compartments within the skin; when melanoma cells progressed through each compartment (or "Clark level"), the likelihood of distant dissemination increased.

Melanoma cells are restricted to the epidermis at:

Level 1: Melanoma in situ.

Level 2: Invasion of solitary melanoma cells or extremely tiny nests into the papillary dermis.

Level 3: Melanoma cells "fill and expand" the papillary dermis at the third stage.

Level 4: Invasion of the dermal reticular layer.

Level 5: Invasion into the subcutaneous fat layer.

Some pathologists still include the Clark levels in their melanoma reports because of the information they provide about the risk of disease aggressiveness, but in 1970, Alexander Breslow independently developed a more accurate method for classifying melanoma based on a measured depth of invasion that captured the thickness of the tumor. Breslow's depth classification system was based on the depth of invasion in millimeters rather than the depth by anatomic compartments, which vary in thickness at different anatomic sites.

Breslow initially classified melanoma into five stages:

Stage I: a thickness of less than or equal to 0.75 mm.

0.76–1.5 mm for Stage II.

1.51–2.25 mm in Stage III.

2.26–3.0 mm in Stage IV.

Greater than 3.0 mm in Stage V [25].

4. Melanoma detection via noninvasive imaging

Modern scientific advances have enabled the creation of noninvasive imaging methods for the diagnosis of melanoma. The development of mobile apps like SkinVision, UMSkinCheck, and MoleScope has been motivated by a desire to improve patients' access to screenings, lower the financial burden of doing so, and find cancers earlier. Numerous studies, however, have shown that such applications are typically wrong [26]. Three out of four algorithms mistakenly identified as many as 30% of melanomas as low-risk tumors, according to a recent research. The potential for these applications to be a valuable tool in the diagnosis of melanoma would increase significantly if their accuracy could be improved and they were subject to strict regulatory control [27]. Experts warn, however, that patients could be harmed if they put too much faith in these technologies in their current iterations. Until then, consumers should exercise caution when it comes to using these apps for melanoma screening [27].

Some melanomas do not meet the ABCDE rule; thus, you should inform your doctor of any persistent sores, strange bumps or rashes, or changes in your skin or existing moles [28].

The use of immunohistochemistry in the diagnosis of melanoma.

4.1 Clinical indicators

For a melanoma diagnosis to be made, a healthcare provider must first identify a lesion as clinically abnormal before doing a biopsy. After a biopsy of a lesion has been taken, further examination at the microscopic level might be conducted. In many cases, melanoma is identified by highly trained pathologists based on a set of well-established histological hallmarks. Histologic subtypes of melanoma can be difficult to distinguish with traditional hematoxylin and eosin (H&E) staining due to the disease's heterogeneity [29]. Also, melanoma has a number of histological imitators, so telling the two apart can be challenging [30]. Immunohistochemistry (IHC) has also been widely employed to interpret difficult cases as knowledge of the molecular mechanisms behind melanogenesis has increased and molecular biomarkers have been developed to aid in melanoma detection [31]. Because of its accessibility in most laboratories, low cost, high reliability, and high reproducibility, immunohistochemistry (IHC) is the most commonly used ancillary test to aid in the diagnosis of melanoma by pathologists. That is why it is not shocking that IHC has been increasingly popular in the last 20 years for the detection of melanoma [31].

Diagnostic and prognostic melanoma biomarkers can be broken down into two categories: melanocytic markers and proliferative markers [32]. An ambiguous lesion can be traced back to its melanocytic origin by testing it for melanocytic markers, which are proteins involved in melanin synthesis, melanosome biogenesis, or melanocyte differentiation. Contrarily, cell cycle activity in a lesion can be assessed with the help of proliferation markers [30]. Counting mitotic figures (mitosis/mm^2) is now the gold standard for measuring tumor proliferation; however, new studies have shown that immunohistochemistry (IHC) detection of proliferative markers can be a robust biomarker of proliferative activity with prognostic significance [33].

This is especially true in staging systems, where IHC has become increasingly important. If tumor cells are not apparent on H&E during a sentinel lymph node examination, the seventh edition of the AJCC recommends using immunohistochemistry (IHC) to improve the detection of micrometastasis [34]. Under the correct conditions, several melanocytic markers provide compelling evidence for melanocytic origin and melanoma. The antibodies melan-A and melanoma-associated resistance to treatment 1 (MART-1) are both responses to the same antigen (melanoma antigen recognized by T-cells) [35]. Detecting melanoma with MelanA/MART-1 is more sensitive than HMB-45, one of the most widely used melanoma biomarkers [36]. Human melanoma black 45 (HMB-45) is an antibody that recognizes gp100, an antigen expressed in melanocytes (also known as Pmel 17) [36, 37]. Melanin polymerization, melanosome biogenesis, and melanogenesis all involve the protein Gp100. The proteins S100, microphthalmia transcription factor (MITF), tyrosinase, and SOX10 are also considered to be typical melanocytic indicators in the diagnosis of melanoma [38]. Some of the most specific markers are melan-A/MART-1 and HMB-45, both of which are expressed only in melanocytic malignancies and a few other, rare kinds of cancer [39, 40]. The melanocytic marker used in the evaluation of a melanocytic lesion is based on the expected outcome. While sensitive indicators like S100 protein and Sox10 can be utilized by pathologists to identify a potentially malignant melanocytic neoplasm, specific markers can be employed to prove beyond a reasonable doubt that the neoplasm in question derives from melanocytes (although some melanocytic tumors may be missed using only these markers). Both high sensitivity and specificity are required of a melanocytic marker.

However, melanocytic markers cannot reliably distinguish between malignant and benign melanocytic growth since they stain all melanocytes [41].

In addition, a false-negative diagnosis may result from the failure to apply more sensitive markers in the case of some types of melanoma (especially desmoplastic melanomas), which lack expression of the most specific melanocytic markers [42].

4.2 Causes of melanoma

Most experts agree that overexposure to sunlight, especially when young, is a key risk factor for melanoma. Statistics indicate that 86% of melanomas are caused by the sun's ultraviolet (UV) rays. How does sun exposure lead to skin cancer? UV exposure can damage a cell's DNA, resulting in modifications to specific genes that influence how cells grow and divide. The risk for complications arises when your skin's DNA is broken and its cells begin to proliferate.

The World Health Organization has classified ultraviolet radiation from tanning beds as a carcinogen (a substance that causes cancer). The use of tanning beds may be associated with more than 6000 occurrences of melanoma per year in the United States.

Although anybody can acquire melanoma, those with the following conditions have an increased risk of developing the disease:

Personal experience with melanoma.

A history of melanomas in the family

The individual has fair skin, freckles, blonde or red hair, and blue eyes.

Sun exposure to the point of blistering sunburns.

Living near the equator or at a high altitude may increase your exposure to ultraviolet light.

A history of use tanning beds.

Numerous moles, particularly unusual moles.

A compromised immune system.

Melanoma is more prevalent among White people; however, all skin types can be affected. Melanoma is typically found on the palms, soles, and nails of those with darker skin [43–45].

4.3 Melanoma cancer statistics

Melanoma is the 17th most prevalent form of cancer found all over the world.

Melanoma and non-melanoma skin cancers are the most common forms of the disease, respectively. The most frequent non-melanoma malignancies are basal cell carcinoma and squamous cell carcinoma.

Several factors make it particularly difficult to estimate the incidence of skin cancer [46]. There are numerous subtypes of skin cancer, which might complicate data collection. For instance, non-melanoma skin cancer is frequently not recorded by cancer registries, or registrations of this illness are frequently insufficient due to the fact that the majority of cases are successfully treated with surgery or ablation. It is possible that the estimated global incidence of skin cancer is an underestimate due to these reasons.

Melanoma of the skin is the 17th most prevalent cancer in the world. It is the 13th most prevalent cancer in men and the 15th most prevalent cancer in women.

In 2020, there were more than 150,000 new instances of cutaneous melanoma [47]. Australia had the highest non-melanoma skin cancer incidence rate in 2020, followed by New Zealand [48]. Australia had the highest incidence of cutaneous melanoma in 2020, followed by New Zealand. In 2020, New Zealand had the highest melanoma skin cancer mortality rate, followed by Norway. In 2020, Papua New Guinea had the highest non-melanoma skin cancer mortality rate, followed by Namibia [49].

4.4 Melanoma prevention with nutrition

In recent years, there has been a lot of research on dietary factors and/or nutritional aspects that may influence melanoma risk. A vast range of dietary chemicals has been examined. However, just a subset of these will be covered in this review. Many have promised in vitro evidence to back up their potential, and some have been linked to a lower risk of melanoma in epidemiologic studies; nevertheless, data from randomized controlled trials in humans are insufficient. Future research could shed light on the potential involvement of dietary components in melanoma risk reduction.

Vitamin D is a well-studied option for melanoma chemoprevention. Although its primary purpose is to regulate calcium and phosphate balance, vitamin D receptors are found on many cells. It has gained significant interest as a potential preventive or complementary treatment strategy for melanoma and other malignancies [50].

Vitamin E is a class of fat-soluble chemicals that include tocopherols and tocotrienols. Because of its antioxidant effects, it is gaining popularity. Vitamin E has been shown in vitro to inhibit several types of malignant cells, including melanoma cells. Recent research has focused on vitamin E derivatives and their potential anti-melanoma activities [51]. There are numerous fatty acids, including saturated, monounsaturated, polyunsaturated (PFA), and trans-unsaturated fatty acids. Some epidemiologic research suggests that unsaturated fatty acids may reduce the risk of several types of cancer, including melanoma [52]. Nicotinamide, often known as niacinamide, is the vitamin B_3 derivative amide form of nicotinic acid. It is a precursor of nicotinamide adenine dinucleotide (NAD+), a cofactor required for energy production, metabolism, and DNA repair. It has recently attracted interest for its potential to counteract UV-induced immunological suppression [53]. Trace amounts of selenium are found in meat, fish, vegetables, grains, and milk. It has been studied as a potential chemopreventive agent cofactor for glutathione peroxidase and thioredoxin reductase antioxidant enzymes. In vitro inhibits melanoma cell growth dose-dependently, halting the cell cycle at G0/G1. Selenium suppresses tumor metastasis in mouse studies but not tumor growth [54].

4.5 Conclusion

This is easy-to-spread melanoma. This disease is difficult to identify and treat. Understanding how melanomas escape the immune system will improve diagnostic and therapeutic methods. Improved melanoma detection and prognosis are being developed.

IHC is now frequently used to diagnose melanoma. Tissue immunohistochemistry seeks cancer markers. This diagnostic (and prognostic) method has limitations. IHC scoring can be subjective; diagnostic systems involving several biomarkers require precise interpretation criteria and standardization methods to assure repeatability between labs and pathologists. Newer, more objective methods may change melanoma diagnosis. Parallel reaction monitoring (PRM) is a high-resolution, high-precision ion monitoring approach. PRM uses mass spectrometry (MS) to detect peptides with known masses, such as histone PTMs. This method tells MS to fragment and sequence just certain-sized ions. Discovery-based MS approaches are less sensitive. Melanoma treatment has improved with BRAF, CTLA4, and PD1 inhibitors. To tackle secondary resistance, scientists are researching novel medications and pharmacological combinations. Why do certain therapies work and others fail? Biomarkers to predict patient response are needed, so clinicians may stratify patients and generate personalized treatments based on mutational and biomarker profiles. Individualized melanoma treatment improves prognosis and costs. It will reduce bad drug administration and patient suffering. Metastatic melanoma avoided treatment until recently. Scientists are beginning to comprehend the genetic and mechanical roots of the disease, which may lead to a cure.

5. Summary

Melanoma is virulent. It is a heterogeneous, complex condition, making diagnosis and treatment difficult. Understanding melanoma genesis and how melanomas avoid the immune system will lead to improved diagnostic and treatment options. New technologies are being developed to improve melanoma diagnosis and prognosis, improving patient outcomes. In the last 20 years, IHC has been used more to diagnose melanoma. Tissue immunohistochemistry research focuses on developing sensitive and specific cancer biomarkers. This diagnostic (and presumably prognostic) tool has limitations. IHC scoring can be subjective, so establishing diagnostic systems combining many biomarkers requires precise interpretation criteria and standardization methods to assure repeatability between labs and pathologists. IHC is a good approach for recognizing biomarkers, but newer, more objective, and repeatable methods could change melanoma diagnosis. Metastatic melanoma treatment has improved with BRAF, CTLA4, and PD1 inhibitors. Researchers have learned how secondary resistance develops and are developing new medications and drug combinations to produce a more lasting effect. Ongoing research investigates why and how these treatments work. Biomarker development is a priority, so doctors can stratify patients and design more tailored treatments based on mutational and biomarker profiles. Personalized melanoma treatment improves prognosis and reduces treatment costs. Ineffective drugs will not be given, reducing patients suffering from adverse effects.

Metastatic melanoma is a ferocious and deadly disease that avoided therapy until recently. We are beginning to understand the disease's genetic and molecular roots, enabling more effective therapies and hope for a cure.

Author details

Ali Khani Jeihooni[1*], Pooyan Afzali Harsini[2], Gholamreza Imani[3] and Saeed Hamzehie[4]

1 Nutrition Research Center, Department of Public Health, School of Health, Shiraz University of Medical Sciences, Shiraz, Iran

2 Department of Public Health, School of Health, Kermanshah University of Medical Sciences, Kermanshah, Iran

3 Department of Medicine, School of Medicine, Kermanshah University of Medical Sciences, Kermanshah, Iran

4 Internal Medicine Specialist, Department of Medicine, School of Medicine, Kermanshah University of Medical Sciences, Kermanshah, Iran

*Address all correspondence to: khani_1512@yahoo.com

References

[1] Prasad RR et al. Silibinin and non-melanoma skin cancers. Journal of Traditional and Complementary Medicine. 2020;**10**(3):236-244

[2] Charalambides M, et al. A review of Mohs micrographic surgery for skin cancer. Clinical and Experimental Dermatology. 2022;47(5):833-849

[3] Hejmadi M. Introduction to Cancer Biology. United Kingdom: Bookboon; 2014

[4] Guy GP, Ekwueme DU. Years of potential life lost and indirect costs of melanoma and non-melanoma skin cancer. PharmacoEconomics. 2011;**29**(10):863-874

[5] Yu L, Oh C, Shea CR. The treatment of non-melanoma skin cancer with image-guided superficial radiation therapy: An analysis of 2917 invasive and in situ keratinocytic carcinoma lesions. Oncology and Therapy. 2021;**9**(1):153-166

[6] Garbe C et al. The evolving field of Dermato-oncology and the role of dermatologists: Position Paper of the EADO, EADV and Task Forces, EDF, IDS, EBDV–UEMS and EORTC Cutaneous Lymphoma Task Force. Journal of the European Academy of Dermatology and Venereology. 2020;**34**(10):2183-2197

[7] Wong SL et al. Sentinel lymph node biopsy for melanoma: American society of clinical oncology and society of surgical oncology joint clinical practice guideline. Annals of Surgical Oncology. 2012;**19**(11):3313-3324

[8] Das P et al. A review article on melanoma. Journal of Pharmaceutical Sciences and Research. 2016;**8**(2):112

[9] Panda S et al. Clinicopathological study of malignant melanoma in a regional cancer center. Indian Journal of Cancer. 2018;**55**(3):292

[10] Bacchetti T et al. Paraoxonase-2: A potential biomarker for skin cancer aggressiveness. European Journal of Clinical Investigation. 2021;**51**(5):e13452

[11] Soumya R, et al. Advanced earlier melanoma detection algorithm using colour correlogram. In: 2016 International Conference on Communication Systems and Networks (ComNet). IEEE. 2016

[12] Yadav N, Banerjee M. Molecular and genetic response of human skin under ultraviolet radiation. In: Photocarcinogenesis & Photoprotection. United States: Springer; 2018. pp. 15-27

[13] Morgan AM, Lo J, Fisher DE. How does pheomelanin synthesis contribute to melanomagenesis? Two distinct mechanisms could explain the carcinogenicity of pheomelanin synthesis. BioEssays. 2013;**35**(8):672-676

[14] Gray-Schopfer V, Wellbrock C, Marais R. Melanoma biology and new targeted therapy. Nature. 2007;**445**(7130):851-857

[15] Shain AH, Bastian BC. From melanocytes to melanomas. Nature Reviews Cancer. 2016;**16**(6):345-358

[16] Rebecca VW, Sondak VK, Smalley KS. A brief history of melanoma: From mummies to mutations. Melanoma Research. 2012;**22**(2):114

[17] Read J, Wadt KA, Hayward NK. Melanoma genetics. Journal of Medical Genetics. 2016;**53**(1):1-14

[18] Cario M, Taieb A. Isolation and culture of epidermal melanocytes. In: Skin Tissue Engineering. United States: Springer; 2019. pp. 33-46

[19] Sample A, He YY. Mechanisms and prevention of UV-induced melanoma. Photodermatology, Photoimmunology & Photomedicine. 2018;**34**(1):13-24

[20] Chaturvedi SS, Gupta K, Prasad PS. Skin lesion analyser: An efficient seven-way multi-class skin cancer classification using MobileNet. In: International Conference on Advanced Machine Learning Technologies and Applications. United States: Springer; 2020

[21] Mulenga M et al. Epidemiological and histopathological profile of malignant melanoma in Malawi. BMC Clinical Pathology. 2019;**19**(1):1-6

[22] Sembiring E. Skin cancer patients profile at faculty of medicine university of North Sumatera pathology anatomy laboratory and Haji Adam Malik general hospital in the year of 2012-2015. In: IOP Conference Series: Earth and Environmental Science. IOP Publishing; 2018

[23] Tchernev G, Temelkova I. Annually over 9 billion dollars less for one-step melanoma surgery: Sounds good. Journal of Biological Regulators and Homeostatic Agents. 2019;**33**(5):1493-1496

[24] Scolyer RA, Long GV, Thompson JF. Evolving concepts in melanoma classification and their relevance to multidisciplinary melanoma patient care. Molecular Oncology. 2011;**5**(2):124-136

[25] Rawson RV, Scolyer RA. From Breslow to BRAF and immunotherapy: Evolving concepts in melanoma pathogenesis and disease progression and their implications for changing management over the last 50 years. Human Pathology. 2020;**95**:149-160

[26] Rat C et al. Use of smartphones for early detection of melanoma: Systematic review. Journal of Medical Internet Research. 2018;**20**(4):e9392

[27] Wang JV, Chapman LW, Keller MS. Challenges to Smartphone Applications for Melanoma Detection. 2017

[28] Rhodes AR. Public education and cancer of the skin. What do people need to know about melanoma and nonmelanoma skin cancer? Cancer. 1995;**75**(S2):613-636

[29] Le Guellec S et al. Loss of H3K27 trimethylation is not suitable for distinguishing malignant peripheral nerve sheath tumor from melanoma: A study of 387 cases including mimicking lesions. Modern Pathology. 2017;**30**(12):1677-1687

[30] Waqar S et al. Recognizing histopathological simulators of melanoma to avoid misdiagnosis. Cureus. 2022;**14**(6):e26127

[31] Kim RH, Meehan SA. Immunostain use in the diagnosis of melanomas referred to a tertiary medical center: A 15-year retrospective review (2001-2015). Journal of Cutaneous Pathology. 2017;**44**(3):221-227

[32] Hessler M et al. Melanoma biomarkers and their potential application for in vivo diagnostic imaging modalities. International Journal of Molecular Sciences. 2020;**21**(24):9583

[33] Martin-Gorgojo A et al. Dysplastic vs. common naevus-associated vs. de novo melanomas: An observational retrospective study of 1,021 Patients. Acta Dermato-Venereologica. 2018;**98**(6)

[34] Durślewicz J et al. Prognostic significance of MATR3 in stage I and II non-small cell lung cancer patients. Journal of Cancer Research and Clinical Oncology. 2022:1-10

[35] Rohaan MW et al. MART-1 TCR gene-modified peripheral blood T cells for the treatment of metastatic melanoma: A phase I/IIa clinical trial. Immuno-Oncology and Technology. 2022;**15**:100089

[36] Nielsen PS, Riber-Hansen R, Torben Steiniche D. Immunohistochemical double stains against Ki67/MART1 and HMB45/MITF: Promising diagnostic tools in melanocytic lesions. The American Journal of Dermatopathology. 2011;**33**(4):361-370

[37] Eisenstein A et al. Emerging biomarkers in cutaneous melanoma. Molecular Diagnosis & Therapy. 2018;**22**(2):203-218

[38] Saida T. Histogenesis of cutaneous malignant melanoma: The vast majority do not develop from melanocytic nevus but arise de novo as melanoma in situ. The Journal of Dermatology. 2019;**46**(2):80-94

[39] Le L et al. Melanosome biogenesis in the pigmentation of mammalian skin. Integrative and Comparative Biology. 2021;**61**(4):1517-1545

[40] Ohbayashi N, Fukuda M. Recent advances in understanding the molecular basis of melanogenesis in melanocytes. F1000Research. 2020;**9**:5-9

[41] Koh SS, Cassarino DS. Immunohistochemical expression of p16 in melanocytic lesions: An updated review and meta-analysis. Archives of Pathology & Laboratory Medicine. 2018;**142**(7):815-828

[42] Revythis A et al. Unraveling the wide spectrum of melanoma biomarkers. Diagnostics. 2021;**11**(8):1341

[43] Schadendorf D et al. Melanoma. The Lancet. 2018;**392**(10151):971-984

[44] Carr S, Smith C, Wernberg J. Epidemiology and risk factors of melanoma. Surgical Clinics. 2020;**100**(1):1-12

[45] Matthews NH et al. Epidemiology of Melanoma. Exon Publications; 2017. pp. 3-22

[46] Gordon LG et al. Estimated healthcare costs of melanoma and keratinocyte skin cancers in Australia and Aotearoa New Zealand in 2021. International Journal of Environmental Research and Public Health. 2022;**19**(6):3178

[47] Skin cancer statistics. [cited 2022 FEB,20,2022]; Available from: https://www.wcrf.org/cancer-trends/skin-cancer-statistics/

[48] Trenerry C et al. "She'll be right, mate": A mixed methods analysis of skin cancer prevention practices among australian farmers—An at-risk group. International Journal of Environmental Research and Public Health. 2022;**19**(5):2940

[49] Arnold M et al. Global burden of cutaneous melanoma in 2020 and projections to 2040. JAMA Dermatology. 2022;**158**(5):495-503

[50] Nikas IP, Paschou SA, Ryu HS. The role of nicotinamide in cancer chemoprevention and therapy. Biomolecules. 2020;**10**(3):477

[51] Rafeeq H et al. Biochemistry of fat soluble vitamins, sources,

biochemical functions and toxicity. Haya: The Saudi Journal of Life Sciences. 2020;**5**(6):188-196

[52] Yang K, Fung TT, Nan H. An epidemiological review of diet and cutaneous malignant melanomaepidemiology of diet and melanoma. Cancer Epidemiology, Biomarkers & Prevention. 2018;**27**(10):1115-1122

[53] Gasperi V et al. Niacin in the central nervous system: An update of biological aspects and clinical applications. International Journal of Molecular Sciences. 2019;**20**(4):974

[54] Oczkowski M et al. Dietary factors and prostate cancer development, progression, and reduction. Nutrients. 2021;**13**(2):496

Section 2

Epidemiology

Chapter 2

Epidemiology of Melanoma

Kasimu Umar Adoke

Abstract

Melanoma is a malignant tumour that arises from melanocytic cells. The incidence is increasing worldwide in white population where fair skin people receive excessive sun exposure. Although relatively uncommon in Africa-Americans, recent trends show increase incidence in Africa- Americans. Prognosis is affected by histological and clinical factors in addition to site of the lesion. It is a well-established facts that the MAPK signaling pathway is hyper activated in up to 90% of melanomas. The dependence of melanoma on this activated pathway has been exploited successfully in the clinics by selectively inhibiting this pathway mainly the BRAF mutated melanoma, which is mutated in approximately 50% of melanomas, although resistance develop in some cases. The improved understanding of the regulatory pathways of the immune system provides great hope for significant clinical impact in some patients. Antibodies inhibiting CTLA-4 and PD-1/PD-L1 signaling have been developed and approved, as monotherapies or in combination, after showing great improvement in patient survival but show limited efficacy in some patients that develop resistance and adverse effects. Better biomarkers are needed in the future to help select better immunothrapeutic agents with potent efficacy, less side effects and less likelihood to develop resistance.

Keywords: melanoma, targeted therapy, immunotherapy, resistance

1. Introduction

Melanocytes are specialised cells in the body that are responsible for the production of the pigment melanin [1, 2]. The melanin is transported in organelles called melanosomes via the elongated dendrites of the melanocytes and functions as a protective barrier against the harmful ultraviolet (UV) radiation, ultimately avoiding DNA damage [3, 4]. Melanoma is the most lethal form of skin cancer and represent less than 5% of all cutaneous malignancies and if diagnosed early it is associated with favourable outcome. Most instances melanoma is associated with distance metastasis with a dismal survival rate **Figures 1** and **2**. Risk factors for melanoma include family history of melanoma, exposure to ultraviolet radiation, the presence of dysplastic nevus, skin colour, hair colour, eye colour, altitude, latitude, xeroderma pigmentosum, immunosuppression, scars, chemical exposures and Marjolin ulcers [5, 6].

IntechOpen

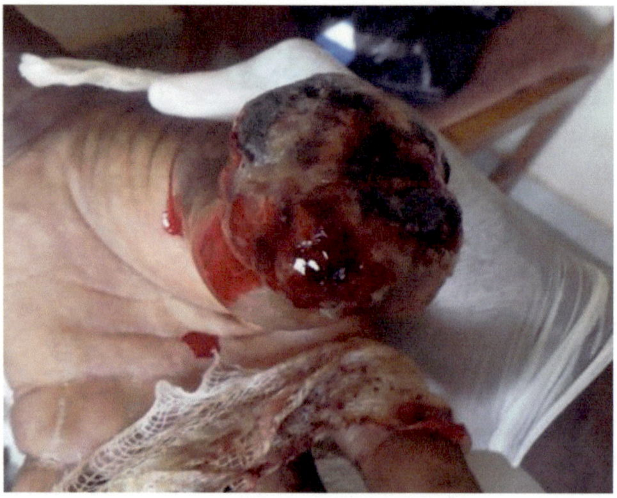

Figure 1.
Subungual melanoma in a 62-year-old male with ulceration.

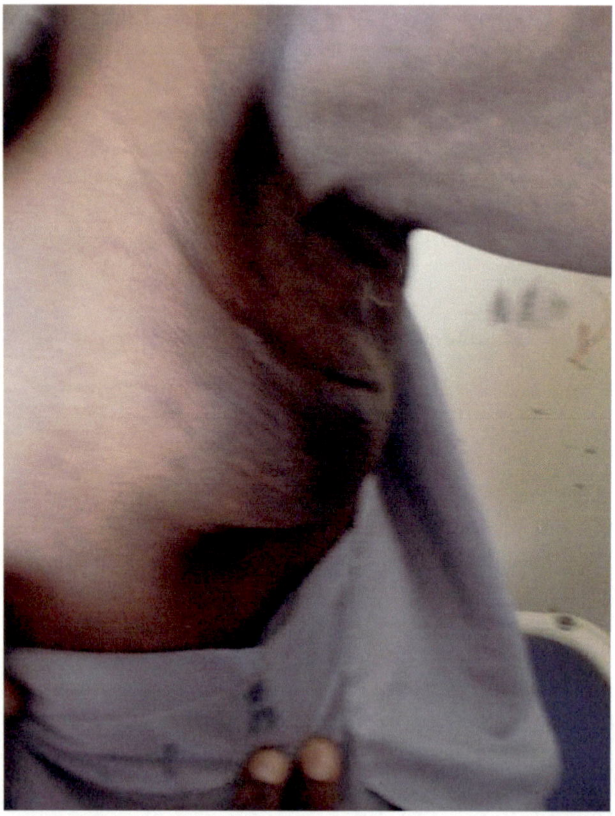

Figure 2.
Metastasis of subungual melanoma to the axillary lymph node in the same patient in **Figure 1**.

2. Incidence

In the last few years, there has been an increased incidence of melanoma in all populations [5]. The incidence rate of cutaneous melanoma is greater in white population groups compared to Hispanic, African-American, Indo-American, and Asian population groups [6]. Increase in incidence rate vary across geographical, ethnicity and gender [7, 8]. The marked differences in the incidence rates are attributed to different pigmentation characteristics that predominate in the populations of different regions, but also to the discrepancy in frequency of recreational sun exposure among countries [9–11]. The annual age-adjusted incidence of malignant melanoma in African American women is approximately 0.7 per 100,000 Although the incidence in Caucasian women and men differs, many reports have found narrow incidence rates between African American women and men (0.7 and 1.0 per 100,000, respectively [12, 13] **Figure 3**. While the incidence of malignant melanoma is not well documented in African populations, the sole of the foot is the commonest site, which has prompted speculations that trauma rather than UV-radiation as etiological factor in African cutaneous melanoma [14]. As in African Americans, acral lentiginous melanoma is the most common type of melanoma found in Asians, with a poor prognosis and 5–10-year survival rates of 80.3% and 67.5%, respectively. Acral lentigenous melanoma is said to occur more in the elderly, commoner on the feet and lacks BRAF mutation. Interestingly, approximately 7.5% of all melanoma in Asians are found in the oral cavity, 60% of which develop from pigmented oral lesions [15]. The superficial spreading melanoma is the most common sub-type representing 70% of melanoma cases (**Table 1**). It can arise denovo in sun exposed areas of the body or in association with a nevus. Nodular melanoma account for 5% of cutaneous melanoma and occurs in the trunk or limbs in the elderly patients with male preponderance. Lentigo maligna melanoma constitutes 4–15% of cutaneous melanoma and correlates with long time sun exposure and increasing age. This lesion affects mostly the head and neck area of the body. Superficial spreading melanoma nearly always arises in white skin individuals and less common in black or brown skin individuals. In a study it constitutes two third of cases of melanoma in Australia and new zealand [16].

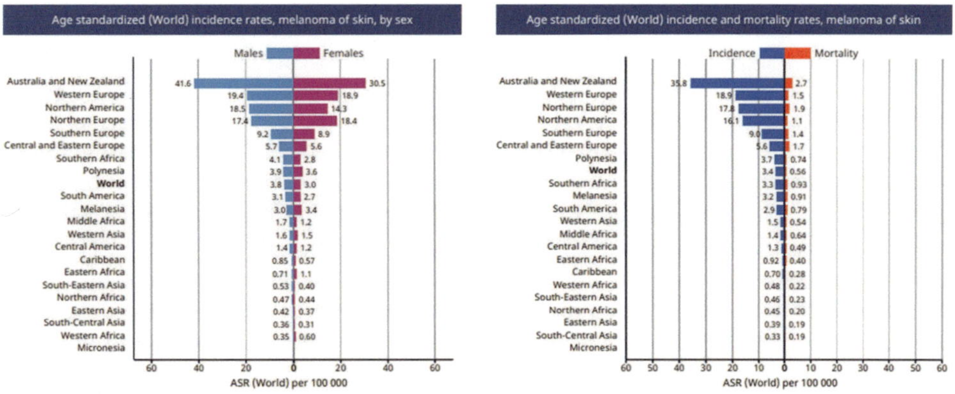

Figure 3.
Melanoma distribution by age and sex (Globocan 2020).

Subtype	Frequency	Characteristic
Superficial spreading	70%	Arises from existing nevus
Nodular	5%	Absence of a radial growth phase, variable presentation and robust vertical invasion
Lentigo Maligna	4–15%	Typically demonstrates slow progression, and frequently appears in sun-exposed areas (i.e., face, head, etc.)
Acral lentiginous	5%	Has higher incidence in patients with darker skin pigmentation and frequently occur on the palms, soles and subungual spaces
Amelanotic	4%	Characterised by absent of pigmentation and considered rare
Desmoplastic	Less than 4%	Rare melanoma seen in older adults that is characterised by scant spindle cells and minimal cellular atypia
Ocular melanoma	Less than 5%	Uveal, conjunctival, blurred vision, visual field defect, can be asymptomatic

Table 1.
Melanoma subtypes.

Mucosal melanomas primarily involve the mucosa of the mouth, anogenital regions, nasal and paranasal sinuses although other mucosal sites can be involved, it has an aggressive course and poor prognosis. It is a rare subtype of melanoma in the Caucasians but it is the second most common subtype in Asians [17]. Mucosal melanoma has a lower mutational burden, a higher rate of NRAS and KIT mutation with low rate of BRAF V600E alterations. Uveal melanoma constitutes less than 5% of all melanomas in the United States and unlike its cutaneous counterpart, it arises from the interstitial melanocytes found abundant in the iris, choroid and ciliary body.

Non-Hispanic white Caucasians have the highest incidence of uveal (5–6) per million and conjunctival melanoma (5–8) per million. The incidence of uveal melanoma in Africans is estimated at (0.3) per million although, the study was mostly derived from African-Americans [18, 19].

3. Risk factors

Studies have shown that people living in geographical areas with increased UV exposure which is inversely correlated with latitude have a higher risk of developing melanoma [20]. Both UVA and UVB are considered carcinogenic to humans but, it is UVB that causes direct damage through formation of pyrimidine dimers while UVA causes DNA damage through production of reactive oxygen species. Melanomas in chronically sun exposed skin tends to have BRAF mutation, inactivation mutation in of NF1, activation mutation in KIT and increase mutational frequency in TP53. In Africa and Asians, cutaneous melanoma is seen in the foot highlighting the fact that trauma could be a causative agent in this region other the UV radiation. Early neonatal exposure to blue-light in cases of hyperbilirubinemia increases the chances of nevi and melanoma [21]. Melanomas can develop in any tissue involved by a nevus and the risk increases with the size and cellularity of the nevus. Familial melanomas have an autosomal dominant pattern of inheritance with high penetrance genes namely CDKN2A and CDK4 [22]. Uveal nevi are well known to transform into uveal melanoma and a minority of families with uveal melanoma carry a germline mutation in the BAP1 (BRCA 1 associated protein-1) gene [23].

4. Melanoma pathways

The mitogen-activated protein kinase (MAPK) pathway are serine-threonine kinases that control cellular pathways such as proliferation, growth, cell transformation and apoptosis hence, plays a critical role in the development of cancers [24]. Mutations in the KRAS, NRAS and KIT have been correlated with the development of melanoma with BRAF V600E seen in almost 50% of melanoma patients, with populations in the US, Brasil, Sweden and Australia correlating to mutations in BRAF melanoma [25]. The activation of this signaling pathway leads to constitutive activation of the mitogen-activated protein kinase (MAPK) pathway that leads to among other thing decrease apoptosis, increase invasiveness and increase metastatic behavior by the tumour cells. KIT gene mutations are present in 39% of mucosal melanomas and 36% of acral lentigenous melanomas with populations in China, Japan, Turkey and Russia [25, 26]. NRAS mutations are found commonly in sun- damaged areas and is present in 20% of melanomas. It's presence correlate with nodular melanoma and with populations in US, Italy, Spain, Sweden [25, 27]. Uveal melanoma carries activation mutation of GNAQ or GNA11 in almost 80% of patients. The genes encode a heterotrimetric GTP-binding protein α- subunit that encodes a G- protein- couple receptor signaling to the MAPK pathway. Mutations in GNAQ has been found in approximately 50% of uveal melanomas while, GNA11 mutations are seen in 32% of uveal melanoma and constitute the commonest mutations seen in metastatic cases. Conjunctival melanomas have BRAF mutations with no GNAQ [28]. Recently, BAP1 has been found in 84% of patients with uveal melanoma and strongly correlates with metastatic behavior in ocular melanoma.

5. Treatment and recent advances

Surgical resection might cure patients with localised primary melanomas, despite surgical resection being the primary treatment option in most malignant melanoma tumours, it is not always enough to reduce the risk of resistance and improve survival. Chemotherapy was the earliest treatment option for advanced-stage melanoma yet, it has proven to be insufficient to improve the overall survival of patients, even when administered in combination with other drugs [29]. Standard chemotherapy for metastatic melanoma is associated with toxicity and in some cases myelosupression. The dependency of melanoma on the MAPK signaling pathways has been exploited successfully by selectively inhibiting this pathway although resistance do develop in some case [30–32]. The genomic landscape of melanoma is also defined by epigenetic changes in complexes of proteins that interact with DNA to regulate gene expression. Development of targeted therapies has been driven by the advanced understanding of the molecular pathways and mechanism of melanoma vis a vis therapy for patients with BRAF V600E mutations has been encouraging with key challenges in some clinical settings. Combination treatment of BRAF with MEK inhibitors have resulted in a better outcome in patients with melanoma, with some having progression free survival of three to six months compared with single therapy with BRAF inhibitors. Recently, the combination of BRAF/MEK inhibitors is used to treat two stages of melanoma namely stage III and IV BRAF mutated melanomas [33, 34]. However, most treated patients will eventually exhibit disease progression due to a constellation of resistance mechanisms emerging from tumor heterogeneity within an individual patient. One of the common strategies of the tumours to develop resistance is to activate the parallel signaling pathway PI3K-AKT-mTOR by activating mutations in PI3KCA or loss of PTEN [34].

During the last decade, the increasing knowledge about the role of the immune system in tumour progression allowed the development of many different immunotherapies. The treatment of advanced melanoma was revolutionised with the development and establishment of immune checkpoint inhibitors (ICIs). Immune checkpoint blockade with anti- cytotoxic T- lymphocyte- associated protein 4 (anti-CTLA-4), anti- programme cell death 1 (anti-PD-1) and its ligand currently form the most effective therapy for metastatic and late stage cutaneous melanoma [35]. Ipilimumab, an anti-CTLA-4 has proven to be effective in T- cell inhibition by tumour cells and activation and proliferation of effector T-cells [36]. Also, Pembrolizumab and nivolumab have shown higher efficacy and less toxicity than ipilimumab [37, 38].

Although cancer immunotherapies have a major impact on patient outcomes, about 60% of patients develop primary resistance, while others experience initial clinical benefit and later on develop secondary resistance. Overall, this highlights the importance of both developing alternative therapeutic strategies to immune check point inhibitors and also identifying better prognostic targets to effectively select patients to undergo a specific type of therapy. Therapies such as intratumoral injection of oncolytic viruses, autologus tumour infiltrating lymphocytes (TIL) and anti-PD-1/anti- LAG have shown promising results in some cases of advanced melanoma.

6. Summary

Melanoma is a highly complex disease comprised of different layers of molecular information, the discovery of additional mutations in human melanomas, as well as strategies for inhibiting their activity, will require continued collaboration between basic and clinical scientists for improved survival and minimised side effects of various therapy.

Acknowledgements

I wish to acknowledge the entire staff of the Department of Pathology, Federal Medical Centre Birnin Kebbi, Nigeria for their assistance toward writing this chapter.

Conflict of interest

I declare no conflict of interest.

Author details

Kasimu Umar Adoke
Federal Medical Centre Birnin Kebbi, Nigeria

*Address all correspondence to: kasimuadoke@gmail.com

References

[1] Brito FC, Kos L. Timeline and distribution of melanocyte precursors in the mouse heart. Pigment Cell & Melanoma Research. 2008;**21**(4):464-470

[2] Mort RL, Jackson IJ, Patton EE. The melanocyte lineage in development and disease. Development. 2015;**142**(4):620-632

[3] Tolleson WH. Human melanocyte biology, toxicology, and pathology. Journal of Environmental Science and Health Part C Environmental Carcinogenesis & Ecotoxicology Reviews. 2005;**23**(2):105-161

[4] Plonka PM, Passeron T, Brenner M, et al. What are melanocytes really doing all day long...? Experimental Dermatology. 2009;**18**(9):799-819

[5] Schneider JS, Moore DH II, Sagebiel RW. Risk factors for melanoma incidence in prospective follow-up. The importance of atypical (dysplastic) nevi. Archives of Dermatology. 1994;**130**:1002-1007

[6] Apalla Z, Nashan D, Weller RB, Castellsagué X. Skin cancer: Epidemiology, disease burden, pathophysiology, diagnosis, and therapeutic approaches. Dermatological Therapy (Heidelb). 2017;**7**:5-19

[7] Cormier JN, Xing Y, Ding M, Lee JE, Mansfield PF, Gershenwald JE, et al. Ethnic differences among patients with cutaneous melanoma. Archives of Internal Medicine. 2006;**166**:1907-1914

[8] Whiteman DC, Green AC, Olsen CM. The growing burden of invasive melanoma: Projections of incidence rates and numbers of new cases in six susceptible populations through 2031. Journal of Investigative Dermatology. 2016;**136**(6):1161-1171

[9] Lee JY, Kapadia SB, Musgrave RH, et al. Neurotropic malignant melanoma occurring in a stable burn scar. Journal of Cutaneous Pathology. 1992;**19**:145-150

[10] Chang AE, Karnell LH, Menck HR. The National Cancer Data Base report on cutaneous and noncutaneous melanoma: A summary of 84,836 cases from the past decade. The American College of Surgeons Commission on Cancer and the American Cancer Society. Cancer. 1998;**83**(8):1664-1678

[11] Ward WH, Farma JM, editors. Cutaneous Melanoma: Etiology and Therapy. Brisbane (AU): Codon Publications; 2017

[12] International Agency for Research on Cancer. Global Cancer Observatory, World Health Organization. Available from: https://gco.iarc.fr/

[13] Cress RD, Holly EA. Incidence of cutaneous melanoma among non-Hispanic whites, Hispanics, Asians, and blacks: An analysis of California cancer registry data,1988-93. Cancer Causes & Control. 1997;**8**:246-252

[14] Baum B, Duarte AM. Skin cancer epidemic in American Hispanic and Latino patients. Pediatrician Skin Color. 2015:453-460

[15] Koh HK. Cutaneous melanoma. The New England Journal of Medicine. 1991;**325**:171

[16] Agbai ON, Buster K, Sanchez M, Hernandez C, Kundu RV, Chiu M. Skin cancer and photoprotection in people of color: A review and recommendations

for physicians and the public. Journal of the American Academy of Dermatology. 2014;**70**:748-762

[17] Richardson A, Fletcher L, Sneyd M, Cox B, Reeder AI. The incidence and thickness of cutaneous malignant melanoma in New Zealand 1994-2004. New Zealand Medical Journal. 2008;**121**(1279):18-26

[18] McLaughlin CC, Wu X-C, Jemal A, et al. Incidence of noncutaneous melanomas in the U.S. Cancer. 2005;**103**:1000-1007

[19] Hu DN, Yu GP, McCormick SA, Schneider S, Finger PT. Population-based incidence of uveal melanoma in various races and ethnic groups. American Journal of Ophthalmology. 2005;**140**(4):612-617

[20] El Ghissassi F, Baan R, Straif K, et al. A review of human carcinogens—Part D: Radiation. The Lancet Oncology. 2009;**10**:751-752

[21] Olah J, Toth-Molnar E, Kemeny L, Csoma Z. Long-term hazards of neonatal blue light phototherapy. British Journal of Dermatology. 2013;**169**:243-249

[22] Hayward NK. Genetics of melanoma predisposition. Oncogene. 2003;**22**:3053-3062

[23] Abdel-Rahman MH, Pilarski R, Cebulla CM, et al. Germline BAP1 mutation predisposes to uveal melanoma, lung adenocarcinoma, meningioma, and other cancers. Medizinische Genetik. 2011;**48**:856-859

[24] Davies H, Bignell GR, Cox C. Mutations of the BRAF gene in human cancer. Nature. 2002;**417**(6892):949-954

[25] Luz DG, John AN, José DT. Differences in mutations in BRAF, NRAS, and KIT in different populations and histological subtype of melanoma: A systemic review. Melanoma Research. 2020;**30**:62-70

[26] Doma V, Barbai T, Beleaua MA, Kovalszky I, Rásó E, Tímár J. KIT mutation incidence and pattern of melanoma in central-east Europe. Pathology Oncology Research. 2020;**26**:17-22

[27] Lito P, Rosen N, Solit DB. Tumor adaptation and resistance to RAF inhibitors. Nature Medicine. 2013;**19**(11):1401-1409

[28] Van Raamsdonk CD, Griewank KG, Crosby MB, Garrido MC, Vemula S, et al. Mutations in *GNA11* in uveal melanoma. The New England Journal of Medicine. 2010;**363**:2191-2199

[29] Batus M, Waheed S, Ruby C. Optimal management of metastatic melanoma: Current strategies and future directions. American Journal of Clinical Dermatology. 2013;**14**(3):179-194

[30] Thompson JF, Scolyer RA, Kefford RF. Cutaneous melanoma. Lancet. 2005;**365**(9460):687-701

[31] Hout FE, Haydu LE, Murali R. Prognostic importance of the extent of ulceration in patients with clinically localized cutaneous melanoma. Annals of Surgery. 2012;**255**(6):1165-1170

[32] Wilson MA, Schuchter LM. Chemotherapy for melanoma. Cancer Treatment and Research Communications. 2016;**167**:209-229

[33] Eroglu Z, Ribas A. Combination therapy with BRAF and MEK inhibitors for melanoma: Latest evidence and place in therapy. Therapeutic Advances in Medical Oncology. 2016;**8**(1):48-56

[34] Rizos H, Menzies AM, Pupo GM. BRAF inhibitor resistance mechanisms in metastatic melanoma: Spectrum and clinical impact. Clinical Cancer Research. 2014;**20**(7):1965-1977

[35] Darvin P, Toor SM, Sasidharan NV. Immune checkpoint inhibitors: Recent progress and potential biomarkers. Experimental & Molecular Medicine. 2018;**50**(12):1-11

[36] Hodi FS, O'Day SJ, McDermott DF. Improved survival with ipilimumab in patients with metastatic melanoma. The New England Journal of Medicine. 2010;**363**(8):711-723

[37] Robert C, Schachter J, Long GV. Pembrolizumab versus Ipilimumab in Advanced Melanoma. The New England Journal of Medicine. 2015;**372**(26):2521-2532

[38] Robert C, Long GV, Brady B. Nivolumab in previously untreated melanoma without BRAF mutation. The New England Journal of Medicine. 2015;**372**(4):320-330

Section 3

Histopathological Characteristics

Chapter 3

Histological Hallmarks of Malignant Melanoma

Gerardo Cazzato, Anna Colagrande, Lucia Lospalluti, Giuseppe Ingravallo, Eliano Cascardi, Miriam Dellino, Saverio Capodiferro, Eugenio Maiorano, Caterina Foti and Leonardo Resta

Abstract

The histopathological diagnosis of malignant melanoma remains the gold standard to allow the patient to access the entire process of the diagnostic-therapeutic-assistance path. Despite the continuous search for markers that can assist in the diagnostic process, there are cases that remain complex to diagnose, and the presence of different criteria among dermatopathologists further complicates the issue. This section will focus on the state of the art of dermatopathological diagnostics of melanoma, starting from the morphological bases up to the latest acquisitions of immunohistochemistry for diagnostic purposes, and molecular biology for therapeutic purposes. Furthermore, we will focus on particularly "challenging" MM histotypes and on what are the current guidelines for a correct diagnosis.

Keywords: malignant melanoma, histopathology, skin, immunohistochemistry, diagnosis

1. Introduction

Malignant melanoma (MM) is known in the medical literature as the "Great Mime" of pathological anatomy, as it can simulate, in different ways, other neoplasms, both of an epithelial nature and of a mesenchymal nature [1]. From the point of view of the location, MM may originate de novo on healthy skin or represent the malignant transformation of a preexisting melanocytic nevus [2, 3]. In the vast majority of cases, MM represents a sporadic event, while in less than 10% it is linked to alterations of tumor suppressor genes (encoded by the chromosomal region 9p21) and shows a hereditary character, for this reason, it is defined as "familial" [4]. Histopathologically, the MM of the skin and/or mucous membranes consists of neoplastic melanocytic elements, fused or epithelioid, with the presence of atypia and, often, mitotic figures. An accurate histological diagnosis is the basis for a clinical management of the patient affected by MM since all the histopathological parameters

IntechOpen

reported in the report have important implications not only from a diagnostic but also from a prognostic point of view.

2. Histological report of malignant melanoma

In the first instance, it is very important to determine whether the lesion we are analyzing constitutes an MM and is properly differentiated from atypical pigmented lesions that can closely simulate MM [5]. Morphologically the cutaneous MM can be classified into four histological subtypes such as superficial spreading type, lentigo maligna, acral lentiginous, and nodular type. If at first we tended to think that this was a mere histological description, in fact, more recent studies have correlated (sometimes very exhaustively) histological subtypes with particular molecular signatures of MM. For example, you can easily appreciate from the last WHO blue book "Classification of Skin Tumour"2018, IARC, that melanomas on skin chronically exposed to the sun have different chromosomal aberration patterns than melanomas that arise on skin with intermittent exposure to ultraviolet (UV) rays or in areas of acral skin or mucous membranes. Therefore, a correct histological recognition of the MM subtype is of great importance and must always be reported in the pathological report of an MM [6].

Figure 1 shows an example of MM with features consistent with "Spitzoid" MM. Note that the lesion is composed of nests of melanocytes with some mitotic figures; top left is possible to appreciate pagetoid spreading of single melanocytes (another useful clue to diagnosis of MM).

Thickness according to Breslow is the strongest and most reliable prognostic factor in MM and is defined as the measurement of the vertical thickness of the neoplasm [7]. The American Joint Committee on Cancer (AJCC) 8th Edition criteria for staging accurately predict sentinel lymph node positivity in clinically melanoma-negative lymph node patients. In fact, when grouped by AJCC cutting points, there was an increased incidence of positive sentinel lymph nodes with increasing tumor thickness: 4% in melanomas below 1.00 mm, 12% in melanomas 1.01–2.00 mm, 28% in melanomas 2.01–4.00 mm and 44% in melanomas over 4.00 mm [8]. But it is important to consider that there are, however, cases in which the thickness of Breslow does not impact perfectly on the prognosis: it is the case of thin melanomas that are able not only to metastasize but also to bring the subject to death with some ease [9]. By

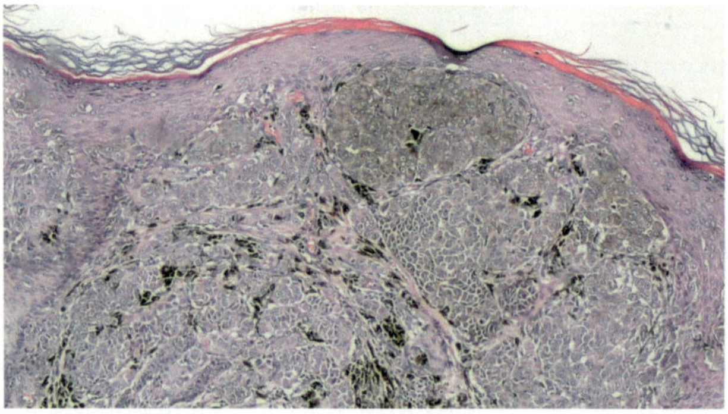

Figure 1.
Histological photomicrograph showing an example of MM (Haematoxylin-Eosin, Original Magnification 10×).

convention, the thickness of Breslow is measured from the granulous layer to the last cell of MM, except in the case of ulcerated lesions, where the base of the ulceration is taken as a reference to the last point where the neoplasm is evident [10].

A parameter related to the thickness of Breslow is the Clark level, which, unlike the first, is a topographical criterion, which is based simply on the definition of which area of skin is affected by MM: superficial (or papillary) dermis, reticular, and subcutaneous. In recent years, the low reproducibility and repeatability of this parameter, due to its rather "subjective" nature of measurement, has in fact caused its disuse, until it is no longer considered mandatory to be included in a histopathological report of melanoma. However, we still consider it correct to include this finding in the MM report as an additional indicator parameter, never to be substituted for Breslow [11].

Another important element that can never be missing in the description of a melanoma is the number of mitoses/mmq. In fact, various studies have shown how the number of mitoses can be a rather reliable indicator of the biological behavior of a given MM (staging and prognosis). Although there is no universally accepted method for counting mitotic figures in melanoma, the AJCC 8′Edition recommends making this measurement in the "hot spot" areas of the lesion, so as to ensure a faithful count of the maximum number of mitoses present in Ref [12].

It is very important to consider one parameter on which there is still no precise agreement in the literature, which is the regression of melanoma. In fact, among the various theories, the most accredited considers the regression as a result of aggression of melanoma cells by the immune system with the substitution of the same with fibrosis, melanophages, lymphocytic infiltrate, and angiectasis. Regression phenomena can be from focal to extended until the complete disappearance of the primary lesion (so-called "burn-out melanoma"). The difficulty of reproducibility of this parameter consists in the variability of what is considered as regression: some studies have considered regression as the total absence of melanoma cells, whereas other studies have also considered more or less partial regression areas in the measurement of regression proper [13]. Regression is now considered to be an independent prognostic factor for worsening prognosis, and according to the College of American Pathologists (CAP) guidelines, regression is measured by a cutoff at 75% [14].

An integral part of a histological report of MM is the evaluation of ulceration, considered an independent prognostic factor for survival associated with melanoma. Ulceration is defined as a continuous "true" solution at full thickness, of the epidermis, with the presence of fibrin deposition or neutrophil granulocytes, and/or reactive hyperplasia of the surrounding epidermis in the absence of trauma or surgical manipulation prior to or in progress. In recent years, more and more evidence supports the need to express the radial extent of ulceration (in mm), as it would seem that more extensive ulcerations correspond to reduced survival values. It should also be remembered that it is necessary to be sure of the presence or absence of this parameter, as over-staging of the MM in question can affect the entire diagnostic-therapeutic-care path of the patient [15].

Lymph vascular invasion (LVI) is a very useful parameter in predicting possible disease diffusion in a metastatic setting. For example, now included in the AJCC 8′Edition, this parameter has been shown to significantly increase the risk of recurrence, lymph node involvement, distant metastases, and death, just like the ulceration parameter [16]. From a histopathological point of view, consideration should be given to the possibility that tissue artifacts can simulate and/or obscure the morphology of lymphatic and/or blood vessels, and, therefore, studies have been carried out [17], which have shown that the use of immunomarkers such as D2–40 (Podoplanin) can help to evaluate true lymph-vascular permeations that could otherwise give false-negatives.

Perineural invasion (PNI) is defined as the infiltration of nerve fibers by melanoma cells, resulting in an extension of the tumor along the surrounding nerves. This parameter is of some importance and should be included in the histological report of the MM, as it (from the literature examined) [18] is a pejorative prognostic factor. In addition, it is good to remember that there are some types of melanoma that are more easily neurotropic, such as desmoplastic melanoma or fused cell melanoma, and, therefore, this aspect is to be considered when diagnosing one of these types of lesions. Indeed, the high local recurrence rate of desmoplastic or fused-cell melanoma requires more aggressive surgery to reduce this risk [19].

Microsatellites are defined in the current CAP recommendations as microscopic and discontinuous cutaneous and/or subcutaneous metastases having a diameter larger or equal to 0.05 mm in the largest dimension, adjacent to a primary melanoma [14]. The presence of microsatellites increases from 4.6% in tumors less than 1.5 mm to 65% in those greater than 4 mm [20]. Furthermore, microsatellites are also associated with an increased frequency of regional lymph node metastasis in tumors greater than 1.5 mm [5, 20].

Lymphocytes infiltrating the tumor (TILs) are a type of lymphocytes capable of attacking neoplastic cells and, depending on the mode and distribution, are divided in ascending order into: absent, non-brisk, or brisk [14]. Several studies tend to point out that an increase in TLLs would be more correlated to an improvement in survival, but also in this area (similar to what we have seen for regression) inter-observer variability does not help to obtain a clearer concordance of studies.

3. Subtypes of malignant melanoma

Melanoma can be considered in the radial growth phase (when melanomatous cells grow in the horizontal plane without giving rise to a vertical growth phase) and in the vertical growth phase, in turn, divisible into tumorigenic (nests/cases deeper than the surface) or non-tumorigenic (melanocytes that do not form a net lesion). It is also very important to consider that melanoma in situ (by definition limited to the basal membrane, therefore, pTis according to AJCC 8′Edition) is different from melanoma in a radial growth phase that, if not called "in situ," suggests the possibility of the presence of some melanocyte minutes present below the basal membrane (c.d. microinvasive).

3.1 Superficial spreading type melanoma (SSM)

Superficial spreading melanoma is the most frequent histotype in the Caucasian population (70–80% of all melanomas). Usually, it is localized to the back in men and to the lower limbs in women. It is the most common type of melanoma in patients with dysplastic nevus syndrome, with familial melanoma and multiple melanomas. Histologically it is characterized, in the intraepidermal component of the horizontal growth phase, by the presence of pagetoid cells (**Figure 2**) and by a proliferation, in the dermal area, of neoplastic cells frequently associated with epitheliod type often to other cytotypes. In many cases, it can observe a horizontal intraepithelial proliferation of the dysplastic nevus type. Atypical cells in single or in small nests can

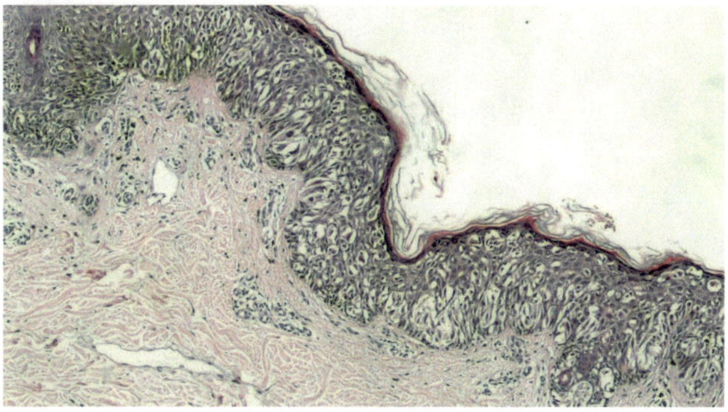

Figure 2.
Histological photomicrograph that shows the features of pagetoid spreading, a major criteria for diagnosing MM (Haematoxylin-Eosin, Original Magnification 10×).

be observed throughout the thickness of the epidermis arranged in an irregular way up to the most superficial layers. In the beginning, the phase of horizontal growth is characterized by invasion of the papillary dermis by single cells or small cell nests. Parallel to the initial invasion, the appearance of a marked inflammatory lymphocytic reaction can be noted. There may be scattered macrophages mixed with inflammatory infiltrate, fibroplasia, and vascular neogenesis. The atypical cells present in the most superficial portion of the papillary dermis, in the horizontal growth phase, have the same cytological characteristics as the cells present in the epidermis, and also the nests of cells are similar in size to those present in the epidermis. In the horizontal growth phase, no cell nest is present in the dermal area, it presents prevailing characteristics compared to the other nests adjacent. The cells of the vertical component, on the other hand, have different cytological characteristics and are predominantly epithelioid-type cells aggregated in nests with cohesive characters. Often a prevailing and expansive type of growth with a tendency for cell proliferation is necessary to develop in a centrifugal direction. The nests of atypical cells, which form the vertical growth, are in size greater than intraepithelial ones. The nuclei are bulky, hyperchromatic, and polymorphic with prominent nucleoli and irregular nuclear membranes. An always evident feature is the lack of cellular maturation with cells with identical cytological features both in the most superficial portion and in the deepest portion of the vertical phase. Mitoses can be in number variable, sometimes even numerous, but above all mitosis is also present in the plus portion of deep melanoma. Isolated cells or groups of necrosing cells are often seen in the dermal component [21, 22].

3.2 Acral lentiginous melanoma (ALM)

ALM is defined as the presence of a horizontal proliferative component characterized by a proliferation of atypical melanocytes, often with dendritic aspects, mainly localized to the basal layer of the epidermis and extended to the skin appendages associated with a lentiginous appearance with a marked elongation of the spurs epithelial (**Figure 3**). The vertical proliferative component is characterized by a proliferation of atypical melanocytes often type epithelioid, spindle, or polymorphic; sometimes the cells can be arranged in bundles such as to simulate a Schwannian differentiation. More frequently it affects the plantar skin and the palmar skin, especially that of the thumb [23].

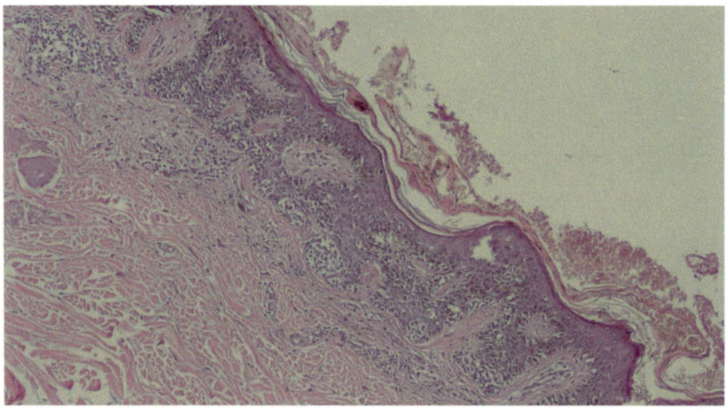

Figure 3.
Photomicrograph showing acral lentiginous MM with the characteristic disposition of melanocytes at the dermo-epidermal junction, with some aspects of pagetoid spreading (Haematoxylin-Eosin, Original Magnificaton 10×).

3.3 Nodular melanoma (NM)

The term nodular melanoma defines a tumor characterized by the appearance of a nodule that develops rapidly without a preexisting phase of horizontal growth (**Figure 4**). Nodular melanoma appears on apparently normal skin. Although no lesion is observed existing or a horizontal phase, however, there may be evidence of an association with a preexisting nevus. Nodular melanoma accounts for about 10–12% of all types of melanoma in Caucasian subjects. This neoplasm is, by definition, already growing vertically, is usually diagnosed at a fairly advanced stage, and has a worse prognosis than other melanomas [24].

3.4 Lentigo maligna melanoma (LMM)

LMM occurs most frequently on the face and sun-exposed upper extremities of elderly people. Macroscopically, there is great variation in color, with tan-brown, black, and even pink areas present. LMM can become an invasive malignancy (vertical growth phase) and it is characterized by thickening of the lesion with the development of elevated plaques or discrete nodules [25]. Histologically, LMM is characterized by an epidermal component of atypical melanocytes, singly and in nests, usually confined to the basal layer and with a little pagetoid invasion of the epidermis (**Figure 5**) [26].

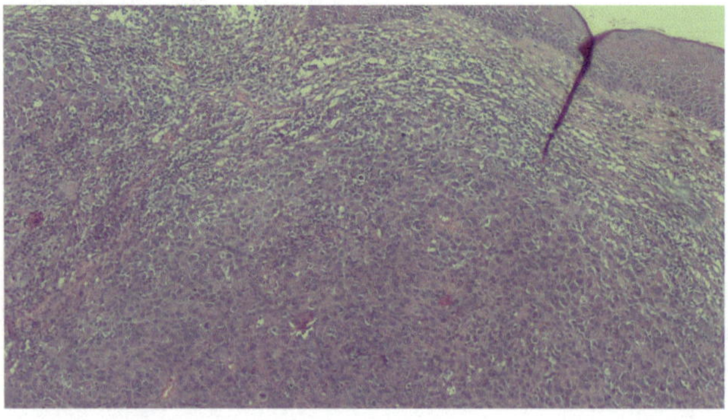

Figure 4.
Example of nodular melanoma (Haematoxylin-Eosin, Original Magnification 10×).

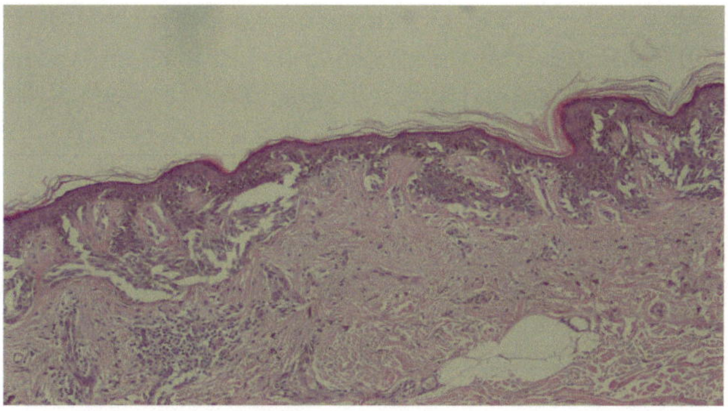

Figure 5.
LMM characterized by some atypical melanocytes that conglomerate in a few atypical nests (Haematoxylin-Eosin, Original Magnification 10×).

4. Other histotypes of MM

4.1 Desmoplastic melanoma (DM)

DM is properly recognized as a variant of MM, with its distinct histological, immunophenotypic, and molecular characterization. The injury is usually considered "scar-like" because, often, the first impression you have at low (panoramic) magnification of this injury is that of a scar. At higher magnification, it is possible to recognize fused cells, immersed in a desmoplastic stroma and focal with myxoid aspects, endowed with mild cytological characteristics, even if at times presenting a "random" pleomorphism (**Figure 6**). Rather characteristically DM cells are quite rich in mast cells and have a tendency to infiltrate the surrounding nerves. This variant of MM prefers the head/neck of older subjects, thus disproving it as a high cumulative solar damage (H-CSD)-related melanoma. Molecular studies have also confirmed a much higher rate of mutations for this lesion histotype than common MM variants [27].

4.2 Nevoid melanoma (NM)

Nevoid melanoma is classically referred to as the "tomb" of the dermatopathologist for its intrinsic ability, even in the eyes of a dermatopathologist with years of

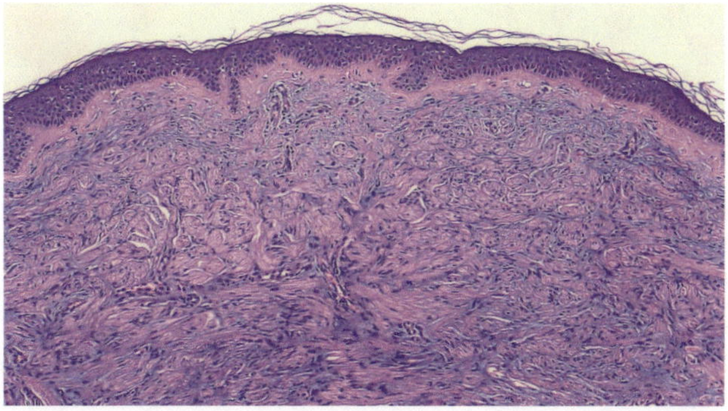

Figure 6.
Histological photomicrograph showing a bland-appereance proliferation that reveals a DM (Haematoxylin-Eosin, Original Magnification 10×).

experience, to mimic a benign melanocytic nevus and, therefore, to pass as unknown. It is a rare type of MM, representing no more than 1% of all melanomas, which is commonly more frequent between the fourth and fifth decades of life, without a gender predominance. Clinically, NM presents as a slowly growing lesion, most commonly on the proximal extremities, trunk, neck, and head [28].

From a histological point of view, NM has an architectural pattern that looks very similar to that of a compound or intradermal nevus, with almost complete symmetry, good circumscription, and minimal or no pagetoid spreading. The most important morphological characteristic distinguishing an NM from a standard nevus is the presence of a monomorphic population of small nevus-like melanic cells, present both in the superficial and deep portions of the dermis. It is of absolute and indispensable importance to conduct a very careful research of mitotic figures, able to make us suspect that we are in front of an NM [29].

5. Immunohistochemical features of malignant melanoma

Melan-A/MART-1 is one of the most important markers of melanocytic differentiation, used in the dermatopathological field. This protein is expressed by melanoma cells and recognized by cytotoxic T cells. Its application is mainly intended for the differential diagnosis of melanocytic tumors, but also for particular other types of tumors, including metastatic since it is more sensitive than another marker, Human Melanoma Black-45 (HMB-45) [30].

HMB-45 is a monoclonal antibody that reacts with an antigen present in melanocytic tumors such as melanomas, hence it is full name of Human Melanoma Black. It is known in pathological anatomy as the best diagnostic marker for melanomas. HMB-45 was discovered in 1986 by doctors Allen M. Gown and Arthur M. Vogel and from then on, its diffusion has become widespread. The specific antigen recognized by HMB-45 is Pmel 17 and reacting positively to melanocytic tumors but not to others is configured for its high specificity and sensitivity.

Despite its high sensitivity HMB-45 has some negative aspects. HMB-45 can be detected only in 50–70% of melanomas. It does not react well to intradermal nevi, normal melanocytes of adult life, fused cell melanoma, and desmoplastic melanoma.

HMB-45 does not react to most malignant tumors that are not melanomas, except for tumors that show melanogenesis (example: pigmented schwannoma, clear-cell sarcoma, or tumors associated with the tuberous sclerosis complex (angiomyolipoma and lymphangiomyoma) [31].

S100 proteins are a family of low molecular weight proteins found in vertebrates, characterized by two binding sites for calcium with helix-loop-helix (EF-hand) structure. There are at least 21 types of S100 proteins and their name "S100" derives from the 100% solubility of these in ammonium sulfate at neutral pH. Most S100 have a homodimeric structure, that is, two identical polypeptides bound together by non-covalent bonds. Although S100 proteins are structurally similar to calmodulins, they differ from these in that they are cell-specific, expressed in particular cells at different levels depending on environmental factors. The calmodulins, on the other hand, are ubiquitous and universal Ca2+ receptors, present in many cells. S100 proteins are normally present in neural crest-derived cells (Schwann cells, melanocytes, and glia cells), chondrocytes, adipocytes, myoepithelial cells, macrophages, Langerhans cells, and dendritic cells.

S100 proteins are implicated in various intracellular and extracellular functions. They are also involved in the regulation of protein phosphorylation, transcription factors, Ca++ homeostasis, the dynamics of cytoskeleton constituents, enzyme activities, cell growth and differentiation, and the inflammatory response. Some members of the S100 family are useful as markers for certain tumors and for the differentiation of cells in the epidermal sense. They can be found in melanomas, malignant peripheral nerve sheath tumors, schwannomas, paraganglioma stromal cells, and clear cell sarcomas [32].

p16 belongs to the family of CDKI, proteins that have the function of inhibiting the action of cyclin-dependent kinase (CDK) and then block the cell cycle. The function of p16 as an inhibitor of cyclin-dependent kinases configures it as a tumor suppressor gene since in its absence it is minus negative control over cell proliferation. It is currently considered another reliable but indicative parameter in differential diagnostics of ambiguous melanocytic lesions [33].

Finally, PRAME (preferentially expressed antigen in melanoma) is a tumor-associated antigen that was first identified through analysis of the specificity of tumor-reactive T-cell clones derived from a patient with metastatic cutaneous melanoma. It was subsequently found that PRAME is not only expressed in cutaneous melanoma but also in ocular melanoma and various nonmelanocytic malignant neoplasms, including non-small cell lung cancer, breast carcinoma, renal cell carcinoma, ovarian carcinoma, leukemia, synovial sarcoma, and myxoid liposarcoma. Normal healthy tissues are not known to express PRAME except for testis, ovary, placenta, adrenals, and endometrium. Because of its expression profile, PRAME is a member of the family of cancer-testis antigens (CTA) and an attractive target for immunotherapy. A number of clinical trials are underway trying to exploit CTAs, including PRAME, for cancer treatment [34]. Although at the beginning there were high expectations of this marker in the dermatopathological diagnosis of malignant melanoma, in reality, with the development of the first studies and the first more numerous cases, the possibility that PRAME can be another indicator within other markers and the always essential morphology has been increasingly outlined, but that its positivity or negativity does not confirm and/or exclude a given diagnosis.

In recent years, there has been an increasing interest in the study of the microenvironment of MM [35]. Research has, in fact, led to the acquisition of new information about cells in the immune system that can control and potentially destroy cancer cells [36]. In this way, it was possible to study how T cells (labeled by the antibody anti-CD4 and/or CD8) were more or less capable of performing their own immunosurveillance functions. It has been possible, therefore, to find that the immune systems are able (as demonstrated earlier in other forms of cancer) to express a receptor, programmed cell death protein 1 or PD1, that binds its ligand called programmed cell death protein 1 ligand or PDL1, going to inhibit the functions of T lymphocyte cells against neoplastic cells [37]. These findings made it possible to formulate pharmacological principles that are known as Immunotherapy. Currently, in 2022, several adjuvant therapies in MM in clinical stage III-IV are considered unresectable. For example, it is important to mention the drug nivolumab, anti-PD1, which by blocking this receptor on T cells, prevents its inhibition mediated by PDL-1 binding and, therefore, enhances the antitumor response of the immune system [38].

6. Next generation sequencing in diagnosis of malignant melanoma

In recent years, the advent of next-generation sequencing (NGS) has made important contributions in the field of pathology, and of neoplasms in general, but also, therefore, in the field of MM [39]. In the case of MM, NGS allowed to highlight molecular alterations that had not previously been discovered, or confirmed, and which had the merit of allowing a greater ability to develop drugs capable of targeting them (for example BRAF) [40]. Although they are mainly used for cancer therapy purposes, NGS can, in some selected cases, also contribute during the diagnostic workout of MM. It is not uncommon, as mentioned above, that the dermatopathological diagnosis of MM is challenging, complex, and not always adequately reachable. For this reason, molecular confirmation of a possible mutation for BRAF can further support a given diagnostic hypothesis, while recognizing that there are cases in which NGS are not of certain diagnostic aid [41].

7. Mucosal melanoma

The mucosal melanoma occurs in the mucosa (mouth, vagina, penis, and conjunctiva) and presents with a quite large, irregularly pigmented macula, representing the growth phase horizontal and with a corresponding nodule or plaque to the vertical growth phase [42]. From the macroscopic point of view, the macular component usually has irregular edges and fairly regular color, but sometimes with a set of brown and brown and bluish-black shades. Sometimes due to the presence of regression, areas of gray-whitish color are noted. The invasive component of vertical proliferation is characterized by a bluish-black nodule but if it is amelanotic it may appear red or whitish-pinkish [43]. From a histological point of view, in addition to the proliferation of uniformly atypical melanocytes placed close to each other along the junction dermo-epidermal, sometimes with elements with evident dendritic extensions, we can observe the presence of invasion by single cells or small nests. Single cells are often fusiform and may be erroneously interpreted as fibroblasts, especially in oral and vaginal seats. Melanoma presents an infiltrate inflammatory scattered, this aspect can be confused with an inflammatory lesion especially if there are macrophages without evidence of pigment. As soon as the proliferation begins vertical, begin to appear more voluminous nests of cells with cytological characters different from those of the proliferative component cells horizontal. Epithelioid cells may be noted as rather large or fused cells and sometimes the vertical component can assume characters desmoplastic. Neurotropism may be present with or without evidence of desmoplasia. These melanomas are almost never associated with or superimposed on a preexisting nevus [44].

Conflict of interest

The authors declare no conflict of interest.

Notes/thanks/other declarations

In memory of Antonietta Cimmino (A.C.).

Author details

Gerardo Cazzato[1*], Anna Colagrande[1], Lucia Lospalluti[2], Giuseppe Ingravallo[1], Eliano Cascardi[1,3], Miriam Dellino[4], Saverio Capodiferro[5], Eugenio Maiorano[1], Caterina Foti[2] and Leonardo Resta[1]

1 Section of Pathology, Department of Emergency and Organ Transplantation (DETO), University of Bari "Aldo Moro", Bari, Italy

2 Section of Dermatology and Venereology, Department of Biomedical Sciences and Human Oncology (DIMO), University of Bari "Aldo Moro", Bari, Italy

3 Unit of Pathology, Candiolo Cancer Institute, Candiolo, Italy

4 Section of Gynecology and Obstetrics, Department of Biomedical Sciences and Human Oncology (DIMO), University of Bari "Aldo Moro", Bari, Italy

5 Department of Interdisciplinary Medicine, University of Bari "Aldo Moro", Bari, Italy

*Address all correspondence to: gerardo.cazzato@uniba.it

References

[1] Cazzato G, Colagrande A, Cimmino A, Demarco A, Lospalluti L, Arezzo F, et al. The great mime: Three cases of melanoma with carcinoid-like and paraganglioma-like pattern with emphasis on differential diagnosis. Dermatopathology (Basel). 2021;**8**(2):130-134

[2] Rosendahl CO, Grant-Kels JM, Que SK. Dysplastic nevus: Fact and fiction. Journal of the American Academy of Dermatology. 2015;**73**(3):507-512. DOI: 10.1016/j.jaad.2015.04.029

[3] Gandini S, Sera F, Cattaruzza MS, Pasquini P, Abeni D, Boyle P, et al. Meta-analysis of risk factors for cutaneous melanoma: I. Common and atypical naevi. European Journal of Cancer. 2005;**41**(1):28-44

[4] Hemminki K, Zhang H, Czene K. Familial and attributable risks in cutaneous melanoma: Effects of proband and age. The Journal of Investigative Dermatology. 2003;**120**(2):217-223

[5] Plaza JA, Prieto VG. Pathology of Pigmented Skin Lesions. New York City: Springer; 2017

[6] WHO Classification of Skin Tumours. WHO Classification of Tumours. 4th ed. Geneve: WHO.

[7] Boada A, Tejera-Vaquerizo A, Requena C, Manrique-Silva E, Traves V, Nagore E. Association between melanoma thickness and clinical and demographic characteristics. European Journal of Dermatology. 2021;**31**:514-520

[8] Keung EZ, Gershenwald JE. The eighth edition American Joint Committee on Cancer (AJCC) melanoma staging system: Implications for melanoma treatment and care. Expert Review of Anticancer Therapy. 2018;**18**(8):775-784

[9] Elder DE. Thin melanoma. Archives of Pathology & Laboratory Medicine. 2011;**135**(3):342-346

[10] Ge L, Vilain RE, Lo S, Aivazian K, Scolyer RA, Thompson JF. Breslow thickness measurements of melanomas around American Joint Committee on Cancer staging cut-off points: Imprecision and terminal digit Bias have important implications for staging and patient management. Annals of Surgical Oncology. 2016;**23**(8):2658-2663

[11] Lyth J, Hansson J, Ingvar C, Månsson-Brahme E, Naredi P, Stierner U, et al. Prognostic subclassifications of T1 cutaneous melanomas based on ulceration, tumour thickness and Clark's level of invasion: Results of a population-based study from the Swedish Melanoma Register. The British Journal of Dermatology. 2013;**168**(4):779-786

[12] Available from: https://www.facs.org/media/jydly2ru/melanoma-8th-ed.pdf. [Accessed: June 23, 2022]

[13] Paredes BE. Regression beim Melanom. Definition, Atiopathogenese, Morphologie und Differenzialdiagnose [Regression in malignant melanoma. Definition, etiopathogenesis, morphology and differential diagnosis]. Pathologe. 2007;**28**(6):453-463

[14] Available from: https://documents.cap.org/protocols/Skin.Melanoma_4.3.0.0.REL_CAPCP.pdf. [Accessed: June 23, 2022]

[15] Eggermont AM, Spatz A, Lazar V, Robert C. Is ulceration in cutaneous melanoma just a prognostic and

predictive factor or is ulcerated melanoma a distinct biologic entity? Current Opinion in Oncology. 2012;**24**(2):137-140

[16] Kashani-Sabet M, Sagebiel RW, Ferreira CM, Nosrati M, Miller JR 3rd. Vascular involvement in the prognosis of primary cutaneous melanoma. Archives of Dermatology. 2001;**137**(9):1169-1173

[17] Petersson F, Diwan AH, Ivan D, Gershenwald JE, Johnson MM, Harrell R, et al. Immunohistochemical detection of lymphovascular invasion with D2-40 in melanoma correlates with sentinel lymph node status, metastasis and survival. Journal of Cutaneous Pathology. 2009;**36**:1157-1163

[18] Quinn MJ, Crotty KA, Thompson JF, Coates AS, O'Brien CJ, McCarthy WH. Desmoplastic and desmoplastic neurotropic melanoma: Experience with 280 patients. Cancer. 1998;**83**(6):1128-1135

[19] Lin D, Kashani-Sabet M, McCalmont T, Singer MI. Neurotropic melanoma invading the inferior alveolar nerve. Journal of the American Academy of Dermatology. 2005;**53**(2 Suppl 1): S120-S122

[20] Karakousis GC, Gimotty PA, Leong SP, Pockaj BA, White RL, O'Donoghue C, et al. Microsatellitosis in patients with melanoma. Annals of Surgical Oncology. 2019;**26**(1):33-41

[21] Situm M, Buljan M, Kolić M, Vučić M. Melanoma--clinical, dermatoscopical, and histopathological morphological characteristics. Acta Dermatovenerologica Croatica. 2014;**22**(1):1-12

[22] Carli P, De Giorgi V, Palli D, Maurichi A, Mulas P, Orlandi C, et al. Patterns of detection of superficial spreading and nodular-type melanoma: A multicenter Italian study. Dermatologic Surgery. 2004;**30**:1371-1375

[23] Goydos JS, Shoen SL. Acral Lentiginous Melanoma. Cancer Treatment and Research. 2016;**167**:321-329

[24] Weiler L, Thomas L, Dalle S. Mélanome nodulaire pigmenté [Pigmented nodular melanoma]. Annals of Dermatology and Venereology. 2013;**140**:827-828

[25] Patterson JW. Weedon's Skin Pathology. Amsterdam: Elselvier; 2020

[26] DeWane ME, Kelsey A, Oliviero M, Rabinovitz H, Grant-Kels JM. Melanoma on chronically sun-damaged skin: Lentigo maligna and desmoplastic melanoma. Journal of the American Academy of Dermatology. 2019;**81**(3):823-833

[27] Nicolson NG, Han D. Desmoplastic melanoma. Journal of Surgical Oncology. 2019;**119**(2):208-215

[28] Diwan AH, Lazar AJ. Nevoid melanoma. Surgical Pathological and Clinical. 2009;**2**(3):521-533

[29] Mesbah Ardakani N, Singh S, Thomas C, Van Vliet C, Harvey NT, Calonje JE, et al. Mitotically active nevus and Nevoid melanoma: A clinicopathological and molecular study. The American Journal of Dermatopathology. 2021;**43**(3):182-190

[30] Busam KJ, Jungbluth AA. A new melanocytic differentiation marker. Advances in Anatomic Pathology. 1999;**6**(1):12-18

[31] Smoller BR, McNutt NS, Hsu A. HMB-45 recognizes stimulated

melanocytes. Journal of Cutaneous Pathology. 1989;**16**(2):49-53

[32] Ohsie SJ, Sarantopoulos GP, Cochran AJ, Binder SW. Immunohistochemical characteristics of melanoma. Journal of Cutaneous Pathology. 2008;**35**(5):433-444

[33] Available from: https://snlg.iss.it/wp-content/uploads/2022/04/LG-411-SIAPEC-IAP.pdf. [Accessed: June 24, 2022]

[34] Lezcano C, Jungbluth AA, Nehal KS, Hollmann TJ, Busam KJ. PRAME expression in melanocytic tumors. The American Journal of Surgical Pathology. 2018;**42**(11): 1456-1465. DOI: 10.1097/PAS.0000000000001134

[35] Neubert NJ, Schmittnaegel M, Bordry N, Nassiri S, Wald N, Martignier C, et al. T cell-induced CSF1 promotes melanoma resistance to PD1 blockade. Science Translational Medicine. 2018;**11**(10):436

[36] Ralli M, Botticelli A, Visconti IC, Angeletti D, Fiore M, Marchetti P, et al. Immunotherapy in the treatment of metastatic melanoma: Current knowledge and future directions. Journal of Immunology Research. 2020;**2020**:9235638

[37] Weiss SA, Wolchok JD, Sznol M. Immunotherapy of melanoma: Facts and hopes. Clinical Cancer Research. 2019;**25**:5191

[38] Larkin J, Chiarion-Sileni V, Gonzalez R, Grob JJ, Rutkowski P, Lao CD, et al. Five-year survival with combined nivolumab and ipilimumab in advanced melanoma. The New England Journal of Medicine. 2019;**381**(16):1535-1546

[39] Serratì S, De Summa S, Pilato B, Petriella D, Lacalamita R, Tommasi S, et al. Next-generation sequencing: Advances and applications in cancer diagnosis. Oncotargets and Therapy. 2016;**9**:7355-7365

[40] Reiman A, Kikuchi H, Scocchia D, Smith P, Tsang YW, Snead D, et al. Validation of an NGS mutation detection panel for melanoma. BMC Cancer. 2017;**17**(1):150

[41] Luo Y, Zhang Z, Liu J, Li L, Xu X, Yao X, et al. Characterizations of gene alterations in melanoma patients from Chinese population. BioMed Research International. 2020;**2020**:6096814

[42] Yde SS, Sjoegren P, Heje M, Stolle LB. Mucosal melanoma: A literature review. Current Oncology Reports. 2018;**20**(3):28

[43] Olla D, Neumeister MW. Mucosal melanoma. Clinics in Plastic Surgery. 2021;**48**(4):707-711

[44] Lerner BA, Stewart LA, Horowitz DP, Carvajal RD. Mucosal melanoma: New insights and therapeutic options for a unique and aggressive disease. Oncology (Williston Park, N.Y.). 2017;**31**:e23-e32

Chapter 4

The Value of Histopathological Characteristics and BRAF and NRAS Mutations for the Diagnosis, Risk Stratification, and Prognosis of Malignant Invasive Melanoma

Tatjana Zablocka and Sergejs Isajevs

Abstract

In recent years, the direction of personalized medicine, which is based on a disease-specific targeting therapy, as well as the early diagnosis of tumors and the identification of high-risk individuals, is rapidly developing in the world. Invasive melanoma is a tumor with high impact for its rapidly growing incidence, high mortality, increased complexity, and high care costs in advanced stages. Recent studies demonstrated the significant value of both conventional histopathological characteristics and genetic alterations in melanoma. This review focuses on the value of conventional histopathological characteristics including histological tumor subtype, Clark level, Breslow thickness, solar elastosis, ulceration, regression, lymphovascular invasion, mitotic counts, peritumoral lymphocyte infiltration, clinical characteristics such as age, gender, length of follow-up after surgery, recurrence, or metastasis, and progression-free survival, and tumor BRAF and NRAS mutations.

Keywords: melanoma, histopathology, tumor infiltration lymphocytes, BRAF, NRAS

1. Introduction

More than 97% of all melanomas are diagnosed with a known primary site, most often on the skin [1–3]. Melanoma can also present within the eye or in the mucosae of internal organs [3]. In the rare cases in which it is diagnosed without an obvious primary site, it is referred to as melanoma of unknown primary (MUP) [3]. The predominant hypothesis to explain MUP involves the spontaneous regression of melanoma from a known primary site [3]. Metastatic melanoma could develop synchronously with a subclinical or otherwise unrecognized cutaneous, ocular, or mucosal melanoma.

Ultraviolet (UV) radiation is the most significant risk factor in the pathogenesis of melanoma, directly damaging DNA [1–3]. Multiple somatic and epigenetic alterations have also been implicated in the pathogenic process, along with the immune response and disturbances of immune tolerance [3].

There is a little evidence for early detection and risk stratification in malignant melanoma [4, 5]. The gold standard for melanoma diagnosis is still histopathological examination of tissues. Histopathological diagnosis involving the qualitative and quantitative assessment of biomarkers is susceptible to substantial interobserver variability, limiting its usefulness for individual patients. Specialized dermatopathologists are likely to be more consistent; however, their expertise is not widely available. Therefore, the standardization of the assessment is important [3].

Deep learning, an automated approach using labeled images to train a network with no other assumptions, has proven useful in many similar areas of digital pathology. In recent years, significant progress has been made in proteomics, metabolomics, and genomics. However, histopathological examination remains the gold standard for the diagnosis and prognosis of melanoma [3, 5–7].

The current World Health Organization (WHO) classification of skin tumors subdivides melanoma on the basis of solar elastosis assessed by dermal elastic fibers to measure cumulative sun damage (CSD) [3]. According to this WHO classification, there are currently three classes of melanomas: those associated with high CSD, those associated with low CSD, and those associated with nodular melanomas [3]. Solar elastosis is usually apparent in superficially spreading melanoma and lentigo maligna melanoma, the so-called high CSD melanoma. Desmoplastic melanoma is associated with increased solar elastosis. The most common subtype of high CSD melanoma is superficially spreading melanoma, which usually begins with early radial growth, followed by vertical growth and invasion of the dermis.

Acral, mucosal, uveal, and spitzoid melanomas are not associated with CSD or are characterized by low CSD. Nodular melanoma usually characterized as a low CSD type with early progression to vertical growth [3].

The development of melanoma is closely related to somatic and epigenetic changes. Different mutations have been implicated in its pathogenesis and evolution. Recent genomic classification subdivides melanoma into four subtypes based on the pattern of the most prevalent significantly mutated genes: BRAF, RAS and NF1 mutants, and triple-WT (wild type) [3, 5].

BRAF, CDKN2, and NRAS mutations are the most important and clinically relevant. The advent of novel personalized treatment for melanoma based on BRAF inhibitors and immunotherapy has reduced the mortality rate over the last decade, but advanced and metastatic melanomas remain difficult to treat [8–10]. Immune tolerance mechanisms are also important in the progression of melanoma.

Germline mutations in the cyclin-dependent kinase inhibitor 2A gene (CDKN2A) are frequently identified in familial melanoma; in 20–50% of such cases, three or more family members are diagnosed with melanoma [11]. Germline mutations in CDKN2A have also been associated with familial atypical multiple mole melanoma (FAMMM) syndrome, an autosomally dominant condition exemplified by a family history of melanoma and large numbers of atypical nevi [3, 11],

Immune responses are important in the pathogenesis of melanoma. Programmed cell death protein 1 ligand 1 (PDL1) and PDL2 are usually expressed by melanoma cells, T cells, B cells, and natural killer cells. This observation led to the development of specific antibodies against programmed cell death protein 1 (PD1) for the personalized treatment of melanoma (for example, nivolumab and pembrolizumab). Combinations of different targeting treatments that influence immune response mechanisms had beneficial effects on melanoma treatment, including PDL1 and CTLA4 targeting and immunotherapy with oncolytic viruses [8–12].

Clinicopathological characteristics, such as tumor size, tumor type, tumor invasiveness (Breslow thickness, Clark level, lymphovascular invasion, and neurotropisms), ulceration, and tumor mitotic activity, are significant prognostic factors for the development and progression of melanoma [3, 11]. In addition, it has been demonstrated that tumor-infiltrating lymphocytes can stratify melanoma into low- and high-risk progression types [13–15].

Diagnostic and therapeutic molecular markers have been increasingly used to assist in the histopathological assessment of melanoma [16]. These markers are helpful not only for diagnosing the condition, but also for distinguishing certain subtypes that could otherwise be difficult to identify [17–24]. BRAF-mutated melanoma is mostly associated with superficial spreading melanoma, younger patients, and non-CSD skin, whereas NRAS mutational melanoma is a nodular subtype associated with CSD skin [20, 25].

Generally, NRAS mutations are independent of BRAF mutations, but dual expression has been reported [25]. The association of NRAS mutations with the degree of solar elastosis suggests that NRAS is closely related to the mutations induced by UV irradiation. Previous studies showed that NRAS mutation is also associated with decreased immune responses in peritumoral melanoma tissue and a more advanced tumor stage [26]. However, the prognostic value of NRAS mutation is still controversial, especially in early-stage melanoma.

1.1 Histopathological assessment of melanoma

At present, the histopathological examination of melanoma is based on the current WHO classification and the College of American Pathologists (CAP) guidelines [3]. Such criteria as tumor type, ulceration, peritumoral lymphocytes, Clark invasion level, Breslow invasion level, lymphovascular invasion, neurotropism, regression, and mitotic activity are routinely assessed. In addition, the excision lines and distance from the tumor are recorded. The pathological tumor node metastasis (pTNM) staging is determined on the basis of histopathological assessment. **Table 1** summarizes the histopathological characteristics for assessing invasive melanoma.

Since Breslow thickness is of particular importance for TNM staging, digital slide analysis could provide better evidence for the measurement of invasions, especially in borderline cases. During recent years, digital pathology has been extensively used not only in research but also in clinical practice. Slide digitalization, scanning, and analysis by artificial intelligence have been suggested as a comprehensive tool to help pathologists construct a final report [27].

Figure 1 shows superficial spreading melanoma. The slide was stained with hematoxylin and eosin, magnification ×100. The tumor cells are located in the epidermis and papillary dermis, with moderate cellular pleomorphism, epidermotropism, and asymmetry. There is prominent peritumoral lymphocyte infiltration.

Melanomas with an amelanotic appearance are more difficult to diagnose. Immunohistochemical staining positive for S100, SOX-10, HMB-45, Melan-A, Mart-1, and tyrosinase supports a diagnosis of melanoma [3].

Some melanomas, especially if regressed and metastatic, can cease to express HMB-45, Melan-A, and tyrosinase. In such cases, the immunohistochemical assessment of melanoma is straightforward; usually, only S-100 and vimentin expression is characteristic.

Figure 2A demonstrates S-100 expression in melanoma immunohistochemically. The arrow indicates positively stained cells. Note cytoplasmic biomarker expression.

Characteristics	
Tumor site	Head and neck, arms, back, trunk, limb
Tumor size	
Histological type, Invasive melanoma	Invasive melanoma Superficial spreading melanoma (low-cumulative sun damage (CSD) melanoma) Lentigo maligna melanoma Desmoplastic melanoma Pure desmoplastic melanoma Mixed desmoplastic melanoma Acral melanoma Melanoma arising in a blue nevus (blue nevus-like melanoma) Melanoma arising in a giant congenital nevus Spitz melanoma (malignant Spitz tumor)
Ulceration	Present/Absent
Tumor Regression	Not identified Present, involving less than 75% of lesion Present, involving 75% or more of lesion
Maximum Tumor (Breslow) Thickness	mm
Anatomic (Clark) Level	Clark I-V level
Mitotical activity	Mitoses/mm^2
Solar elastosis	0–3
Microsatellite(s)	Present/Absent
Lymphovascular Invasion	Present/Absent
Neurotropism	Present/Absent
Tumor-Infiltrating Lymphocytes	The lymphocyte distribution score 0 = absence of lymphocytes within the tissue, 1 = presence of lymphocytes occupying <25% of the tissue, 2 = presence of lymphocytes occupying 25 to 50% of the tissue, and 3 = presence of lymphocytes occupying >50% of tissue
Margins	Distance from Invasive Melanoma to Peripheral Margin, mm Distance from Invasive Melanoma to Deep Margin, mmm
Regional lymph nodes status	Total Number of Lymph Nodes Size of Largest Nodal Metastatic Deposit, mm Extranodal involvement Total Number of Lymph Nodes with Tumor Sentinel Lymph Nodes with Tumor
Distant metastasis	Not identified Site
pTNM	

Table 1.
The protocol for routine clinical examination of melanoma.

Figure 2B demonstrates SOX-10 expression in melanoma tissue immunohistochemically. The arrow indicates positively stained cells. Note the positive nuclear staining of melanoma cells.

Recently, it has been shown that p16 expression in melanoma is significantly lower than nevus [28]. PRAME has also been demonstrated as an immunohistochemical marker to aid the diagnosis of malignant melanoma [29].

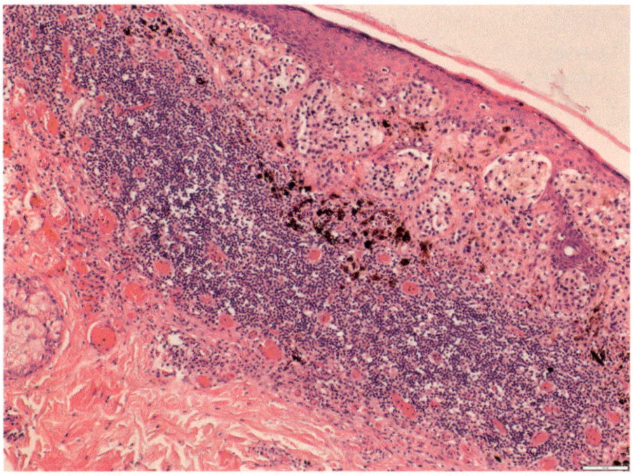

Figure 1.
Representative photomicrograph demonstrated superficial spreading melanoma. Hematoxylin-eosin staining method, magnification: ×100, and scale bar: 20 µm.

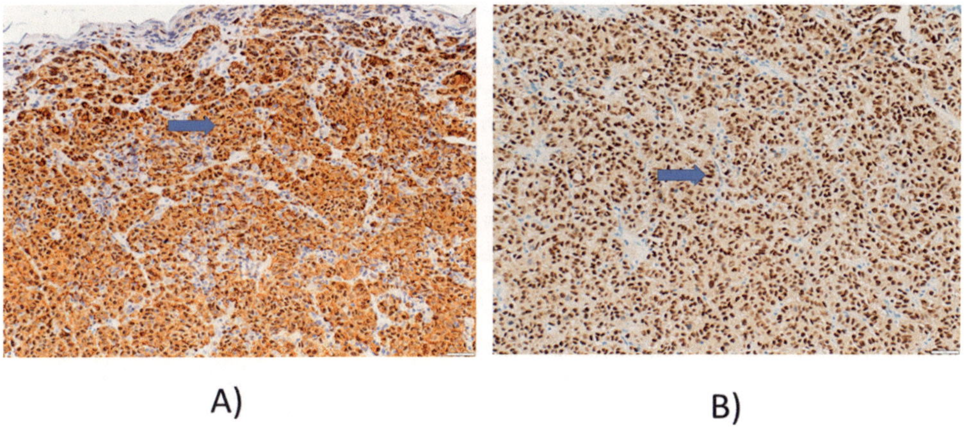

Figure 2.
Representative photomicrograph of biomarker expression melanoma. A. S-100, B. SOX-10. Immunohistochemical staining method, magnification: ×200, and scale bar: 50 µm.

1.2 Artificial intelligence in the histopathological assessment of melanoma

Artificial intelligence (AI) and its subdisciplines of machine learning (ML) and deep learning (DL) are emerging as key technologies in healthcare with the potential to change lives and improve patient outcomes in many areas of medicine. While there is considerable promise for AI technologies in health, there are challenges ahead. These include recognition that it will be extremely difficult for AI to achieve full automation in the diagnostic/clinical pathway. Most efforts to date have focused on the development of neural network architectures to enhance the performance of different computational pathology tasks. U-Net has been used in several applications.

Recently, a deep learning network called MVPNet—multiviewing path deep learning neural networks for magnification invariant diagnosis in breast cancer—has been proposed for the digital analysis of breast cancer. MVPNet has significantly fewer parameters than standard deep learning models and combines local and global features.

During the past decade, advances in precision oncology have resulted in an increased demand for predictive assays that enable patients to be selected and stratified for treatment.

In the global market, there is a high demand for digital pathology and artificial intelligence software for consultations and automated data analysis. Recently, the Food and Drug Administration (FDA) approved the first digital pathology software for automated prostate cancer assessment.

The possibility of digitizing whole-slide images of tissue has led to the advent of artificial intelligence and machine learning tools in digital pathology, which enable subvisual morphometric phenotypes to be mined and could ultimately improve patient management [30].

1.3 Tumor-infiltrating lymphocytes for stratifying the risk of melanoma progression

Tumor-infiltrating lymphocytes (TILs) are considered a manifestation of the host immune response to the tumor [13–15].

Cell membrane-bound antigens different from those of normal cells are characteristic of tumor cells. These antigens are recognized as nonself by antigen-presenting cells, with subsequent activation of cellular and humoral immune responses. The key cells for cytotoxic immune responses are CD4, CD8, and NK cells; for humoral responses, they are B lymphocytes and plasma cells. However, a tumor can escape immune surveillance by unmasking its antigens and inducing apoptosis in the immune cells. The key characteristic of tumor immunity is the presence of peritumoral and intratumoral inflammatory cells. Tumor-infiltrating lymphocytes (TILs) arise from different inflammatory cells, mainly CD4 and CD8 T cells, plus CD20 B lymphocytes and NK cells. These cells have been extensively described in antitumor immunity. T-regulatory lymphocytes, which form the key cell population of peritumoral and intratumoral lymphocytes, have immunoregulatory features. They suppress the immune response and commonly express FOXP3, CD4, and CD25 [13–15].

It has been shown that peritumoral lymphocyte infiltration (TIL) is valuable for melanoma prognosis. It is also closely associated with tumor metastasis to lymph nodes. Patients with increased TIL infiltrate have a better prognosis [13]. Furthermore, increased TIL infiltration is a sign of longer progression-free survival and overall survival, and a lower mortality rate [31].

However, American Joint Committee for Cancer (AJCC) manuals have not included the assessment of TIL for tumor staging and prognosis, and some pathology guidelines do not require peritumoral lymphocyte infiltration to be assessed [3]. The College of American Pathologists (CAP) and the Royal College of Pathologists of Australasia (RCPA) protocols suggest that peritumoral lymphocyte infiltration be assessed as brisk and nonbrisk infiltration. The association of TIL with an improved prognosis for melanoma remains controversial [32–34]. Previous studies have shown that an increased TIL infiltrate is associated with more favorable survival outcomes [13, 30, 31].

A recent study showed that melanoma patients with high TIL grade had significantly better progression-free survival than patients with low TIL grade [15]. The authors recommend incorporating the assessment of TIL into a scoring system, for example from 0 to 3, by estimating the percentage cellular infiltration of the tissue.

The scoring system was defined as follows: 0 = absence of lymphocytes from the tissue, 1 = lymphocytes occupying <25% of the tissue, 2 = lymphocytes occupying 25–50% of the tissue, and 3 = lymphocytes occupying >50% of tissue. Low TIL infiltration was defined as scores of 0 and 1. High TIL infiltration was defined as scores of 2 and 3 [15]. This scoring system correlated significantly with progression-free survival and showed perfect concordance among pathologists; therefore, it could be recommended for routine clinical practice.

1.4 Assessment of BRAF gene mutation for stratifying the risk of melanoma progression

The BRAF gene is located on the seventh chromosome and encodes BRAF protein, one of the signaling kinases in the MAPK pathway. BRAF mutations are the most common genetic alterations in cutaneous melanoma. The prevalence of BRAF mutations among the different melanoma subtypes and populations ranges from 40% to 60% of cases [16–19, 25]. BRAF mutations lead to the constitutive activation of the MAPK pathway. The most common BRAF mutation (80% of all alterations in the gene) is V600E [20]. V600K and V600R mutations are other examples [21].

Previous studies have shown that the BRAF V600E mutation is associated with the superficial spreading melanoma subtype, solar elastosis, younger patients, and melanoma localization on the extremities and back. In contrast, BRAF V600K mutations are correlated with skin sites with high CSD, such as the head and neck, and with older patients [14–19, 35–40].

Recently, whole-genome sequencing of benign melanocytic nevi revealed BRAF mutations in addition to NRAS mutations, the mutational load being positively correlated with UV exposure. The mutational loads in congenital nevi were lower [23].

A recent study revealed associations between BRAF V600 mutational status and younger patient age, Clark invasion level, Breslow thickness, lymphovascular invasion, female gender, and TIL [15].

1.5 Assessment of NRAS gene mutation for stratifying the risk of melanoma progression

The importance of NRAS mutations for the progression of melanoma is controversial. Some studies have shown associations between NRAS mutation and melanoma prognosis, while others found that NRAS mutations have no value for assessing the prognosis [3, 11, 41, 42].

The RAS gene family includes genes that encode the G proteins responsible for cell growth and cell cycle regulation. Three major members of the RAS gene family are NRAS, KRAS, and HRAS. NRAS-mutant melanomas often have dysregulated cell cycles, characterized by the upregulation of cyclin D1 and loss of the tumor suppressor p16INK4A [43].

The NRAS gene is most frequently mutated at hotspots in exon 2 (codons 12 and 13) and exon 3 (codon 61) [42, 44–47]. Mutations of NRAS have previously been associated with the nodular subtype of the primary tumor and localization in sun-damaged skin [45].

Some studies have shown that NRAS mutation is associated with a favorable prognosis [46]. In contrast, others have demonstrated that this mutation is associated with a worse prognosis [48, 49], and some found no significant association at all between NRAS mutation and a prognosis of melanoma [45, 50, 51].

Recent evidence showed that in up to 20–30% of cases, NRAS mutations coexisted with BRAF mutations. Patients with both BRAF and NRAS mutations had worse prognoses than those with BRAF mutant melanoma alone [25, 26]. Since the prognosis for co-mutations is worse, routine NRAS assessment of all the primary melanoma cases would seem to be beneficial.

The assessment of NRAS mutation in melanoma, especially in BRAF-wild-type melanoma, is beneficial since targeted treatment is considered for NRAS mutant melanoma [52]. Immune checkpoint inhibitors (anti-CTLA4 and/or anti-PD1) are the standard treatment in these cases. However, a recent clinical trial also showed promising results from targeted treatments of PI3K-AKT-mTOR, MEK, and CDK4/6.

2. Conclusion

In recent years, the direction of personalized medicine, which is based on disease-specific targeting therapy, along with the early diagnosis of tumors and identification of high-risk individuals, has developed rapidly around the world.

The gold standard for melanoma diagnosis is histopathological investigation and routine evaluation of, e.g., tumor type and tumor invasiveness. Histopathological slide digitalization seems to be beneficial for standardizing the assessment of histopathological characteristics. In addition, the assessment of peritumoral lymphocyte infiltration and BRAF and NRAS mutation status in early-stage melanoma has proved to be of significant value for the risk stratification of disease progression and for personalized treatment.

The assessment of BRAF and NRAS mutations in melanomas is important not only for personalized targeting treatment, but also for prognosis and surveillance strategy. BRAF and NRAS mutations correlate with primary tumor type and disease stage. NRAS mutant melanoma has a significantly worse prognosis than BRAF mutant melanoma, and an active surveillance strategy should be applied to patients with this condition.

Acknowledgements

The study was supported by project "Strengthening of the capacity of doctoral studies at the University of Latvia within the framework of the new doctoral model" identification No. 8.2.2.0/20/I/006. The assistance of BioMedES UK (www.biomedes.biz) in the final drafting of this chapter is acknowledged.

Conflict of interest

The authors declare no conflict of interest.

Author details

Tatjana Zablocka[1,2,3,4*] and Sergejs Isajevs[1,2,4]

1 University of Latvia, Faculty of Medicine, Riga, Latvia

2 Riga East University Hospital, Riga, Latvia

3 Pauls Stradins Clinical University Hospital, Riga, Latvia

4 Hospital of Traumatology and Ortopaedics, Riga, Latvia

*Address all correspondence to: tatjana.zablocka@gmail.com

References

[1] Yang K, ASW O, Slominski RM, Brożyna AA, Slominski AT. Current molecular markers of melanoma and treatment target. International Journal of Molecular Sciences. 2020;**16**:3535

[2] Forsea AM. Melanoma epidemiology and early detection in Europe: Diversity and disparities. Dermatology Practical & Conceptual. 2020;**10**(3):e2020033

[3] Scolyer R, Massi D, Willemze R, Elder DE. WHO Classification of Skin Tumours. WHO, International Agency for Research on Cancer (IARC); 2018

[4] Shellenberger R, Nabhan M. Kakaraparthi S: Melanoma screening: A plan for improving early detection. Annals of Medicine. 2016;**48**:142-148

[5] Mandalà M, Massi D. Tissue prognostic biomarkers in primary cutaneous melanoma. Virchows Archiv. 2014;**464**(3):265-281

[6] Elder DE, Bastian BC, Cree IA, Massi D, Scolyer RA. The 2018 World Health Organization classification of cutaneous, mucosal, and uveal melanoma: Detailed analysis of 9 distinct subtypes defined by their evolutionary pathway. Archives of Pathology & Laboratory Medicine. 2020;**144**:500-522

[7] Fong L. Small EJ anti-cytotoxic T-lymphocyte Antigen-4 antibody: The first in an emerging class of immunomodulatory antibodies for cancer treatment. Journal of Clinical Oncology. 2008;**26**:5275-5283

[8] Hodi FS, O'Day SJ, McDermott DF, Weber RW, Sosman JA, Haanen JB, et al. Improved survival with Ipilimumab in patients with metastatic melanoma. The New England Journal of Medicine. 2010;**363**:711-723

[9] Topalian SL, Sznol M, McDermott DF, Kluger HM, Carvajal RD, Sharfman WH, et al. Survival, durable tumor remission, and Long-term safety in patients with advanced melanoma receiving Nivolumab. Journal of Clinical Oncology. 2014;**32**:1020-1030

[10] Dummer R, Ascierto PA, Gogas HJ, Arance A, Mandala M, Liszkay G, et al. Encorafenib plus Binimetinib versus Vemurafenib or Encorafenib in patients with Braf-mutant melanoma (Columbus): A multicentre, open-label, randomised phase 3 trial. The Lancet Oncology. 2018;**19**:603-615

[11] Bastian BC. The molecular pathology of melanoma: An integrated taxonomy of melanocytic neoplasia. Annual Review of Pathology. 2014;**9**:239-271

[12] Sorokins V, Tilgase A, Olmane E, Isajevs S, Zablocka T, Rasa A, et al. A progressive stage IIIB melanoma treated with oncolytic ECHO-7 virus: A case report. SAGE Open Medical Case Reports. 2020;**8** [eCollection]

[13] Park CK, Kim SK. Clinicopathological significance of intratumoral and peritumoral lymphocytes and lymphocyte score based on the histologic subtypes of cutaneous melanoma. Oncotarget. 2017;**8**(9):14759-14769

[14] Maibach F, Sadozai H, Morteza S, Jafari S, Hunger RE, Schenk M. Tumor-infiltrating lymphocytes and their prognostic value in cutaneous melanoma. Frontiers in Immunology. 2020;**11**:2105

[15] Zablocka T, Nikolajeva A, Kreismane M, Pjanova D, Isajevs S.

Addressing the importance of melanoma tumor-infiltrating lymphocytes in disease progression and clinicopathological characteristics. Molecular and Clinical Oncology. 2021;**15**(6):255

[16] Network CGA. Genomic classification of cutaneous melanoma. Cell. 2015;**161**:1681-1696

[17] Melis C, Rogiers A, Bechter O, van den Oord JJ. Molecular genetic and immunotherapeutic targets in metastatic melanoma. Virchows Archiv. 2017;**471**:281-293

[18] Pracht M, Mogha A, Lespagnol A, Fautrel A, Mouchet N, Le Gall F, et al. Prognostic and predictive values of oncogenic Braf, Nras, C-kit and Mitf in cutaneous and mucous melanoma. Journal of the European Academy of Dermatology and Venereology. 2015;**29**:1530-1538

[19] Ny L, Hernberg M, Nyakas M, Koivunen J, Oddershede L, Yoon M, et al. BRAF mutational status as a prognostic marker for survival in malignant melanoma: A systematic review and meta-analysis. Acta Oncologica. 2020;**59**(7):833-844

[20] Eigentler T, Assi Z, Hassel JC, Heinzerling L, Starz H, Berneburg M, et al. Which melanoma patient carries a BRAF-mutation? A comparison of predictive models. Oncotarget. 2016;**7**(24):36130-36137

[21] Davies H, Bignell GR, Cox C, Stephens P, Edkins S, Clegg S, et al. Mutations of the Braf gene in human cancer. Nature. 2002;**417**:949-954

[22] Long GV, Menzies AM, Nagrial AM, Haydu LE, Hamilton AL, Mann GJ, et al. Prognostic and Clinicopathologic associations of oncogenic Braf in metastatic melanoma. Journal of Clinical Oncology. 2011;**29**:1239-1246

[23] Menzies AM, Haydu LE, Visintin L, Carlino MS, Howle JR, Thompson JF, et al. Distinguishing Clinicopathologic features of patients with V600e and V600k Braf-mutant metastatic melanoma. Clinical Cancer Research. 2012;**18**:3242-3249

[24] Colebatch AJ, Ferguson P, Newell F, Kazakoff SH, Witkowski T, Dobrovic A, et al. Molecular genomic profiling of melanocytic nevi. Journal of Investigative Dermatology. 2019;**139**:1762-1768

[25] Rose EE, Egyhazi S, Omholt K, Mansson-Brahme E, Platz A, Hansson J, et al. NRAS and BRAF mutations in melanoma tumours in relation to clinical characteristics: A study based on mutation screening by pyrosequencing. Melanoma Research. 2006;**6**(6):471-478

[26] Chiappetta C, Proietti I, Soccodato V, Puggioni C, Zaralli R, Pacini L, et al. Braf and Nras mutations are heterogeneous and not mutually exclusive in nodular melanoma. Applied Immunohistochemistry & Molecular Morphology. 2015;**23**:172-177

[27] De Logu F, Ugolini F, Maio V, Simi S, Cossu A, Massi D, et al. Recognition of cutaneous melanoma on digitized histopathological slides via artificial intelligence algorithm. Frontiers in Oncology. 2020;**10**:1559

[28] Milman T, Zhang Q, Ang S, Elder D, Ida CM, Salomao DR, et al. Conjunctival nevi and melanoma: Multiparametric immunohistochemical analysis, including p16, SOX10, HMB45, and Ki-67. Human Pathology. 2020;**103**:107-119

[29] Lezcano C, Jungbluth AA, Busam KJ. PRAME immunohistochemistry as an ancillary test for the assessment of melanocytic lesions. Surgery Pathology Clinical. 2021;**14**(2):165-175

[30] Hekler A, Utikal JS, Enk AH, Berking C, Klode J, Schadendorf D, et al. Pathologist-level classification of histopathological melanoma images with deep neural networks. European Journal of Cancer. 2019;**115**:79-83

[31] Azimi F, Scolyer RA, Rumcheva P, Moncrieff M, Murali R, McCarthy SW, et al. Tumor-infiltrating lymphocyte grade is an independent predictor of sentinel lymph node status and survival in patients with cutaneous melanoma. Journal of Clinical Oncology. 2012;**30**(21):2678-2683

[32] Taylor RC, Patel A, Panageas KS, Busam KJ, Brady MS. Tumor-infiltrating lymphocytes predict sentinel lymph node positivity in patients with cutaneous melanoma. Journal of Clinical Oncology. 2007;**25**(7):869-875

[33] Burton AL, Roach BA, Mays MP, Chen AF, Ginter BA, Vierling AM, et al. Prognostic significance of tumor infiltrating lymphocytes in melanoma. The American Surgeon. 2011;**77**(2):188-192

[34] Mandala M, Imberti GL, Piazzalunga D, Belfiglio M, Labianca R, Barberis M, et al. Clinical and histopathological risk factors to predict sentinel lymph node positivity, disease-free and overall survival in clinical stages I-II AJCC skin melanoma: Outcome analysis from a single-institution prospectively collected database. European Journal of Cancer. 2009;**45**(14):2537-2545

[35] Tas F, Erturk K. Clinical and prognostic significance of BRAF V600E mutation in non-metastatic cutaneous melanoma patients. Neoplasma. 2019;**66**(4):631-636

[36] Bezić J, Kuret S, Vrbičić B, Smolić J, Borić I, Škifić I, et al. Clinicopathological characteristics of BRAF V600E mutated melanomas in the Dalmatian region of Croatia. Acta Dermatovenerologica Croatica. 2019;**27**(4):225-230

[37] Spathis A, Katoulis AC, Damaskou V, Liakou AI, Kottaridi C, Leventakou D, et al. BRAF mutation status in primary, recurrent, and metastatic malignant melanoma and its relation to histopathological parameters. Dermatology Practical & Conceptual. 2019;**9**(1):54-62

[38] Kim SY, Kim SN, Hahn HJ, Lee YW, Choe YB, Ahn KJ. Meta analysis of BRAF mutations and clinicopathologic characteristics in primary melanoma. Journal of the American Academy of Dermatology. 2015;**72**(6):1036-1046.e2

[39] Estrozi B, Machado J, Rodriguez R, Bacchi CE. Clinicopathologic findings and BRAF mutation in cutaneous melanoma in young adults. Applied Immunohistochemistry & Molecular Morphology. 2014;**22**(1):57-64

[40] Aksenenko MB, Kirichenko AK, Ruksha TG. Russian study of morphological prognostic factors characterization in BRAF-mutant cutaneous melanoma. Pathology, Research and Practice. 2015;**211**(7):521-527

[41] Thomas NE, Edmiston SN, Alexander A, Groben PA, Parrish E, Kricker A, et al. Association between Nras and Braf mutational status and melanoma-specific survival among patients with higher-risk primary melanoma. JAMA Oncology. 2015;**1**:359-368

[42] Lee JH, Choi JW, Kim YS. Frequencies of Braf and Nras mutations are different in histological types and sites of origin of cutaneous melanoma: A meta-analysis. The British Journal of Dermatology. 2011;**164**:776-784

[43] Randic T, Kozar I, Margue C, Utikal J, Kreis S. NRAS mutant melanoma: Towards better therapies. Cancer Treatment Reviews. 2021;**99**:102238

[44] Platz A, Egyhazi S, Ringborg U, Hansson J. Human cutaneous melanoma; a review of NRAS and BRAF mutation frequencies in relation to histogenetic subclass and body site. Molecular Oncology. 2008;**1**:395-405

[45] Jakob JA, Bassett RL Jr, Ng CS, Curry JL, Joseph RW, Alvarado GC, et al. NRAS mutation status is an independent prognostic factor in metastatic melanoma. Cancer. 2012;**118**(16):4014-4023

[46] Devitt B, Liu W, Salemi R, Wolfe R, Kelly J, Tzen CY, et al. Clinical outcome and pathological features associated with NRAS mutation in cutaneous melanoma. Pigment Cell & Melanoma Research. 2011;**24**(4):666-672

[47] Ugurel S, Thirumaran RK, Bloethner S, Gast A, Sucker A, Mueller-Berghaus J, et al. B-RAF and N-RAS mutations are preserved during short time in vitro propagation and differentially impact prognosis. PLoS One. 2007;**2**(2):e236

[48] Heppt MV, Siepmann T, Engel J, Schubert-Fritschle G, Eckel R, Mirlach L, et al. Prognostic significance of BRAF and NRAS mutations in melanoma: A German study from routine care. BMC Cancer. 2017;**17**(1):536

[49] Ellerhorst JA, Greene VR, Ekmekcioglu S, Warneke CL, Johnson MM, Cooke CP, et al. Clinical correlates of NRAS and BRAF mutations in primary human melanoma. Clinical Cancer Research. 2011;**17**(2):229-235

[50] Schlaak M, Bajah A, Podewski T, Kreuzberg N, von Bartenwerffer W, Wardelmann E, et al. Assessment of clinical parameters associated with mutational status in metastatic malignant melanoma: A single-Centre investigation of 141 patients. The British Journal of Dermatology. 2013;**168**(4):708-716

[51] Bucheit AD, Syklawer E, Jakob JA, Bassett RL Jr, Curry JL, Gershenwald JE, et al. Clinical characteristics and outcomes with specific BRAF and NRAS mutations in patients with metastatic melanoma. Cancer. 2013;**119**(21):3821-3829

[52] Grimaldi AM, Simeone E, Festino L, Vanella V, Strudel M, Ascierto PA. MEK inhibitors in the treatment of metastatic melanoma and solid tumors. American Journal of Clinical Dermatology. 2017;**18**(6):745-754

Section 4

Surgical Treatment

Chapter 5

Skin Substitutes and Biologic Agents for Wound Closures after Melanoma Resection

Monal Depani and James F. Thornton

Abstract

Wound healing is a highly complex process mediated by microscopic cellular interactions. An improved understanding of the physiology of wound healing has laid the groundwork for translational research to create biologic wound care technologies that have significantly impacted patient care. Biologic wound technologies have broad applications and have had a significant impact on the reconstructive ladder, as the reader will see throughout this chapter. Despite their frequent use, many surgeons are unfamiliar with the plethora of products on the market, as well as each product's relative advantages and disadvantages. This chapter will go over oncologic reconstruction of the nose, scalp, lip, cheek, and extremities after wide local excision of melanomas in these areas, which is a significant challenge for plastic surgeons. Traditional methods for reconstructing these defects include primary closure techniques, skin grafts, local flaps, pedicled flaps, and free tissue transfer; however, the increased risk of metastasis associated with melanoma makes it difficult to use biologic wound healing agents like Integra and Cytal as alternative reconstructive options without causing additional donor site morbidity. In this chapter, we examine the use of biological agents in soft tissue reconstruction, including the surgical approaches, complications, and limitations of various reconstructive methods.

Keywords: plastic surgery, reconstruction, biocompatible materials, acellular dermis, wounds and injuries, lip, cheek, nose, scalp, extremity, melanoma, cutaneous malignancies

1. Introduction

The largest organ in the body, the integument, performs a variety of vital tasks like thermoregulation and defense against environmental microorganisms [1, 2]. Given these roles, injuries to the integument and underlying soft tissue can be anything from merely unsightly to, in the case of severe burns, potentially fatal. Independent of the deformity, the goals of reconstructive surgery are to optimally restore the patient's shape and function. Although there are numerous methods for reconstructing these defects, there are clinical situations where their application is constrained [3]. Several biologic wound care products were created as a result of these challenging situations and developments in our understanding of the physiology of wound healing.

Biological wound agents have advanced the reconstructive ladder since they were originally created in the late 20th century and are now used to repair abnormalities in the skin, soft tissue, and bone [4–6]. The classification of biologic wound care products used in skin and soft tissue restoration, as well as benefits and drawbacks of their application, will be covered in this chapter.

Biologics, biomaterials, and bioconstructs are all names that can be used to refer to a large group of products created from human or animal tissue, or synthetic materials made from organic compounds. As a scaffold for cellular proliferation and differentiation, these substances can be incorporated into or used to replace host tissue as they stimulate wound repair on a cellular level [7–12].

The function, anatomical structure, cellular makeup, and material type are only a few of the features used to categorize biologics [8]. For convenience, we categorize these products based on whether they contain bioactive cells or are acellular in design. Dermoinductive, or cellular, products contain living cells that encourage the creation of extracellular matrix and the growth of new tissue. These cells are often fibroblasts or keratinocytes [13–16]. Products that are dermoconductive or acellular serve as regenerative scaffolds for cell migration, cell proliferation, and the production of extracellular matrix [10]. By enhancing the angiogenic qualities of cytokines generated by the product's cells, dermoinductive wound agents are believed to better aid wound healing when compared to the other types of products [17, 18]. Integra (Integra LifeScience Corporation, Princeton, NJ) and other dermoconductive technologies are believed to be less immunogenic than dermoinductive ones, boosting the success of reconstructive procedures [17, 19]. Several randomized controlled trials comparing cellular and acellular wound agents are ongoing at the time this book was written, but preliminary results indicate that both types of agents are equally effective [17, 19]. In numerous trials, it has been demonstrated that both medicines offer comparable-to-superior results when compared to conventional wound treatment [20–32].

Patients and healthcare professionals have an alternative to conventional reconstructive techniques attributable to the use of biologic wound healing agents in head and neck soft tissue reconstruction [7]. Their effectiveness in challenging surgical situations has received significant acknowledgment [20, 22, 26, 33–36]. These synthetic dermal substitutes, which are useful in a variety of settings, can significantly affect the rates of tissue regeneration and scar development. Notably, they offer a practical answer for covering soft tissue abnormalities resulting from tumor removal.

The final treatment for melanoma resection surgery entails extirpation and thorough dissection to obtain clear margins. Unfortunately, patients may be left with major tissue abnormalities that disrupt the natural symmetry of their face, necessitating reconstructive surgery. Due to restrictions on the surrounding tissue envelope, the severity of the disease's involvement, and cosmetic considerations, reconstructing soft tissue in these areas after melanoma removal presents a considerable challenge for plastic surgeons. Traditional methods for closing these defects include skin grafts, regional flaps, and pedicled flaps; however, developments in skin replacements over the past few decades have produced adaptable substitutes for patients and healthcare professionals [37]. In addition, the development of acellular dermal matrices like Integra (Integra LifeScience Corporation, Princeton, NJ) and Cytal/MicroMatrix (ACell Inc., Columbia, MD) provides solutions for denuded avascular structures. These materials can also be used in conjunction with skin grafting in a staged reconstruction for better skin-tone matching and improved cosmesis [38–41].

1.1 Applications

The surgeon must assess the location, size, and depth of the wound to decide whether the patient will benefit from the use of a biological agent before choosing the best one for them [42, 43]. The surgeon must also assess the defect to see if any underlying tissues, such as tendons, bones, or blood arteries, are exposed. The surgeon must then describe the condition and quality of the wound bed. Although their indications for use have substantially broadened, biologic wound treatments were traditionally used in burn and abdominal wall restoration [43]. Several dermoinductive and dermoconductive wound agents have currently been approved by the United States Food and Drug Association (FDA) for the purpose of soft tissue reconstruction; nevertheless, many reconstructive surgeons use them off-label to fix defects not explicitly permitted by the FDA [44].

2. Scalp reconstruction

The epidermis, dermis, galea aponeurotica, loose areolar tissue, and periosteum—overlying the calvarium—are the five tissue layers that make up the scalp [45]. The epidermis and dermis are composed primarily of fat, adnexal appendages, and hair follicles. The avascular barrier created by the subgaleal loose areolar tissue separates the periosteum's outer layers from its highly vascularized center [45]. The superficial temporal, postauricular, occipital, supraorbital, and supratrochlear branches of the scalp's vascularity are provided by the external and internal carotid arteries [45]. Blood flows inward through these branches to build an intricate network of anastomoses as it moves from the scalp's edges into the center [45]. This offers the best foundation for grafting and the application of dermal substitutes.

Baseline considerations for scalp reconstruction should include the affected region of the scalp, the amenability of the scalp tissue to flap reconstruction, and the healing method. Galeal aponeurosis mobility is constrained by big defects due to its relative rigidity. Compared to the central scalp and vertex, the lateral regions of the galeal aponeurosis typically display more flexibility. Even with relatively bigger defects, the loose areolar tissue can frequently be mobilized to create a flap [45].

Our institution has focused on increasing the use of biologic wound-healing therapies for scalp reconstruction after oncologic resections more recently [46]. Biologic wound-healing agents provide constant, dependable results with high success rates and very few downsides when used in conjunction with color-matched split-thickness skin grafts. Dermal substitute placement is a reasonably simple surgery that can be completed in less than an hour with either local anesthetic or intravenous sedation, drastically reducing on overall operating time. Additionally, there is no additional scar burden because it does not require for the creation of additional incisions. Although there are many dermal substitute products available, Integra is the biologic we favor because it produces the most trustworthy outcomes. Integra was initially just applied to defects requiring bone burring of the calvarium to create deep margins. This restricted its usage in patients with minor defects or intact periosteum. The expanded approach for wound agents allowed us to apply Integra directly to unburred bone in defects less than 4 cm or on the wound beds for all patients with an intact periosteum. Our reasoning for bone burring was further broadened to cover any lesions with dispersed soft tissue, more than 4 cm of exposed bone, any past radiation history, and other questionable soft tissue vascularity.

3. Nasal reconstruction

Given its prominent physical position as the most central part of the face, the nose can significantly contribute to defining a person's overall identity as well as their esthetic look [47, 48]. Therefore, it is crucial that surgeons take into account the delicate foundations of each reconstruction. This necessitates a full comprehension of the intricate nature of nasal anatomy, as well as the value of esthetics for the patient. The superficial fatty layer, fibromuscular layer, and deep fatty layer make up the nasal soft tissue structurally. The superficial musculoaponeurotic system, which is located under the nasal perichondrium and periosteum, serves as the division between the superficial and underlying tissues [49]. When considering the esthetic subunits of the nose: the lower third is made up of the soft triangles, columella, tip, and ala, while the upper two-thirds are confined by the dorsum and nasal sidewalls [50].

Our institution now uses a Depani et al. algorithm to direct the use of biological agents in nasal reconstruction [46]. The strength of these therapies is their capacity to expedite healing without requiring delayed full-thickness skin grafting, which is especially important for reconstructions. Wounds with a properly vascularized bed can be first temporized using Integra or an ACell construct rather than subjecting patients to additional risks including donor-site morbidity and poor color-matching. Then, if necessary, a delayed split- or full-thickness skin graft can be performed; alternatively, patients who are still viable can simply move on to secondary healing. An additional application of ACell to the wound bed can boost the overall effects of the product and raise the likelihood of successful healing. We have been able to considerably enhance outcomes in both upper and lower nasal restorations because of this approach. Our use of biological agents significantly decreased the necessity for distant flap reconstructions for procedures involving the upper nose. Additionally, the dorsum and sidewall's structural characteristics make these agents favorable for satisfactory esthetic results.

The value of biologics was less significant in the lower third of the nose, but our understanding of how they can be used is continually changing. At first, our institution used very few ACell matrices for lower nose reconstructions. Early iterations of

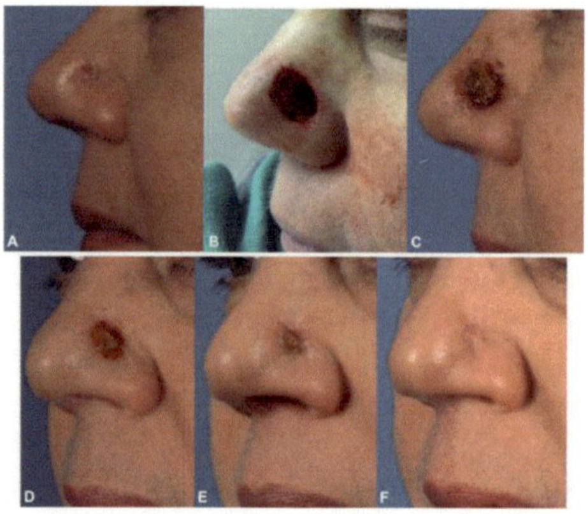

Figure 1.
A 74-year-old female with skin malignancy. (A) Photograph was taken before excisional surgery of the lesion at the left alar groove. (B) Resultant defect involving the left ala and sidewall. (C) 12 days after ACell MicroMatrix and Cytal placement; (D) 30 days postoperatively; (E) 60 days postoperatively; and (F) 4 months postoperatively.

our technique did not believe the use of biologics was necessary; lower nose reconstructions were nearly always closed with flaps due to the anatomic consequences of these surgeries. The sole exceptions to this rule were two patients that were ruled unfit for secondary procedures because the graft bed was not properly vascularized. In these two patients, the necessary vascular basis was established using ACell constructs, facilitating secondary full-thickness grafting (**Figure 1**). Applying an ACell construct made of Cytal and MicroMatrix in these circumstances can lessen the burden of undesirable scarring and eliminate the need for delayed full-thickness skin grafting.

4. Lip reconstruction

The lips are one of the first facial features that people notice during interpersonal interactions, and the ordinary person can immediately detect tiny flaws and distortions [51–53]. The patient can eat, drink, and speak clearly attributable to the lips' ability to control oral competency in addition to their cosmetic value [54]. Furthermore, because they are so important in the display of emotion, the lips are also crucial parts of nonverbal communication. The architecture of the upper lip differs from that of the lower lip in that it has several esthetically significant subunits, such as the philtrum, white roll, and Cupid's bow. The use of biological wound treatments for lip reconstruction comes with a number of challenges. First, because biologic wound agents need a wound bed to integrate with the patient's native tissue, they can only restore partial thickness deficits of the mucosal and cutaneous lip. Second, both deliberate and involuntary motions of the lip can disrupt the interaction between the wound bed and the wound agent. The importance of biologic wound agents for lip reconstruction cannot be understated, despite these drawbacks.

The senior author uses a specific technique to restore mucosal-only defects. In essence, an acellular dermal matrix in sheet form called Cytal Wound Matrix (ACell Inc., Columbia, MD) is sutured over the defect and packed with MicroMatrix (ACell Inc., Columbia, MD), an acellular dermal matrix. After that, patients are told to use Surgilube (HR Pharmaceuticals Inc., York, PA), a water-soluble lubricating jelly, up to five times daily for 3–5 weeks. When compared to local and regional flaps, the reconstructive surgeon can produce outstanding esthetic results with this procedure with little to no lip distortion [55]. It should be noticed that the lip will initially develop dark granulation tissue before it is replaced with mucosa that looks natural. Other acellular dermal matrices have been used with comparable esthetic results to reconstruct vermillion-only lesions [56, 57]. After primary reconstruction, if minor variations still exist, further revisions can be done using autologous fat grafting or fillers.

For reconstructing cutaneous deformities of the lip, biologic wound treatments have a limited role. To prepare the wound bed for subsequent definitive reconstruction with a full-thickness skin graft, dermoconductive wound agents like Integra Bilayer Wound Matrix (Integra LifeSciences, Princeton, NJ) may be employed. Use of biologic wound treatments lowers the chance of scar contracture as compared to skin grafting alone, lowering the danger of distorting nearby structures like the vermilion or, in the case of the upper lip, the nose [58]. MicroMatrix and Cytal Wound Matrix can be used as indicated in the preceding section in place of the Abbe flap when a defect involves the white roll and vermillion.

5. Cheek reconstruction

The ability of the surgeon to reconstruct the defect without producing retraction of the lips, nose, or eyelids is a key factor in successful cheek reconstruction [59, 60]. The reconstructive strategy should take this into consideration because the eyelid, in particular, is more vulnerable to extrinsic stressors. The cheek is divided into three visual zones, each with its own esthetic and practical considerations [61]. Locoregional tissue transfer and skin grafting procedures are the main reconstructive approaches utilized to treat partial thickness defects, regardless of the zone(s) that are affected [62–64]. The reconstructive method for partial thickness cheek defects also includes biological wound agents, but only in specific clinical situations.

A key component of cheek soft tissue reconstruction is the cervicofacial advancement flap [65]. Patients who are unable to discontinue anticoagulant and antiplatelet drugs are not recommended for this surgery because it increases intraoperative complications. It is better to reconstruct the defect with a biologic wound agent with or without delayed skin grafting for patients who lack soft tissue flexibility, such as those who have previously undergone rhytidectomy or who cannot stop taking anticoagulants and antiplatelet treatment. Finally, patients whose surgical specimens are awaiting pathology examination may employ biologic wound agents as a temporary remedy, however this is rarely done in the long-term situation due to the exorbitant cost of these agents.

6. Extremity reconstruction

The most frequent cancers overall are cutaneous malignancies, with UV light being the main risk factor for their occurrence [66]. There is a significant incidence of carcinogenesis on the face, more notably in the H-zone. The lower extremities,

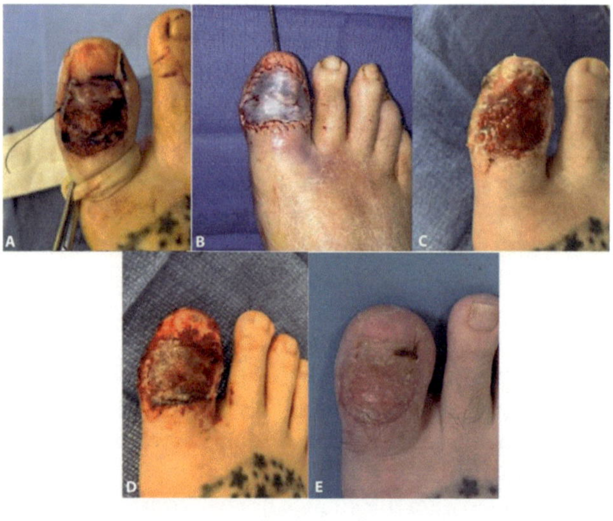

Figure 2.
Use of Integra to reconstruct a post-ablative defect of the great toe following resection of an ungual melanoma in a 72-year-old male. Photograph of post-ablative defect (A), percutaneous pin fixation with Kirshner wire used to stabilize the joint laxity that occurred secondarily to tumor excision (B), 25 days following placement of Integra (C), placement of STSG 25 days after initial excision and placement of Integra (D, E).

which are often in many locations less exposed to the sun, occur less frequently. Both non-melanoma and melanoma skin cancers have the potential to cause localized tissue damage, with the latter having a high chance of metastasizing [67, 68]. Additionally, certain melanomas skin cancers are known for appearing in places that are not exposed to the sun directly, such the soles and subungually [69–71] (**Figure 2**). Extensive local excision is currently the gold standards of therapy for melanoma skin malignancies [72–74]. These resections produce defects that range in complexity and magnitude, and they frequently cause serious functional and psychological impairment in the people who are affected.

Given the lack of surrounding tissue available for reconstruction with local muscle and fasciocutaneous flaps, lesions of the legs and feet can be particularly challenging to reconstruct in comparison to those of the thigh. In addition, numerous lesions expose underlying tendon and bone, especially those that are present in the dorsal side of the foot and the distal third of the leg. Free tissue transfer is frequently regarded as the gold-standard reconstructive technique to address these defects, but if microvascular reconstruction is not an option, biologic wound treatments are a great option [75]. In this chapter, we discuss how soft tissue defects in the lower extremities can be repaired with biological wound treatments after melanoma resections.

The best functional and esthetically pleasing results after reconstructing leg and foot deformities depend on meticulous preoperative planning. The surgeon must take into account the soft tissue quality and laxity of the surrounding area in addition to the defect's location, size, and depth while assessing a defect. The surgeon must take a detailed medical and social history in addition to assessing the wound to find any medical issues or lifestyle choices that might have an adverse effect on the results of reconstructive surgery. Most significantly, people who smoke, have had radiation therapy in the past, or have peripheral artery disease are more likely to experience postoperative problems [76, 77].

Split-thickness skin grafting (STSG) can often be used to reconstruct superficial defects that preserve the underlying muscles, tendons, and bones with acceptable results [76]. However, adding biological wound agents before graft placement is typically beneficial for larger superficial lesions [78]. Biologics followed by STSG have been demonstrated to significantly reduce scar contracture over time, which is consistent with outcomes observed in the care of patients with third-degree burns [79].

On the other hand, defects that expose the underlying tendon or bone require more complicated management. Since the tendons are naturally poorly vascularized, they rely significantly on synovial fluid and the soft tissue that lies above them for hydration, lubrication, and defense against the outside environment [80]. Exposed tendons are more prone to dehydration, which lowers compliance and limits the ability of each muscular contraction and relaxation to move fluidly [81]. On the other hand, although strongly vascularized, bony structures are vulnerable to infection when they are unprotected by soft tissues [82]. Deeper defects that expose the paratenon or periosteum need to be covered surgically, and standard autologous skin grafts cannot be used in these situations.

For both the patient and the surgeon, biologic wound agents have several benefits. First, patients who are medically unfit for extensive microsurgical repair can receive soft tissue coverage in an outpatient environment by using biologic agents [75, 76]. The incidence of medical comorbidities that can lead to unfavorable surgical outcomes is much higher than it would be in the general population because numerous patients having oncoplastic repair of cutaneous malignancies are middle-aged or older [83]. In the event that the size of the soft tissue defect exceeds a certain threshold and the size of the free flap required for reconstruction results in unacceptable levels of donor site morbidity, biologic wound agents may be used. Before final reconstruction with an STSG, small lesions can be easily reconstructed with biologic wound agents in regions where locoregional tissue transfer is challenging, such as the dorsum of the great toe. Acellular dermal matrix products can also be used as a temporary fix until the patient is cleared for permanent reconstruction if the surgical pathology evaluation results are incomplete.

7. Complications and limitations

7.1 Complications

Biologic wound agents are frequently used for wound reconstruction, with different degrees of success. Even though most of these wounds heal adequately after their initial application, problems do occasionally occur [13, 84]. Infection is the most frequent and preventable complication of using biological wound agents [84]. Infections can often be cured with antibiotics and negative pressure wound care early in their clinical course, avoiding the need for surgical intervention [85]. It should be noted that individuals receiving Integra for reconstruction frequently have a creamy exudate at the surgical site between weeks 3 and 5 [86]. Since this phenomenon is sometimes misinterpreted as a soft tissue infection, a thorough evaluation of the patient is necessary to spot any physiologic indications of an infection before beginning an aggressive antibiotic regimen.

Another complication that plastic surgeons face frequently is the biological wound agent detaching and delaminating from the wound bed. To reduce this possibility, it is essential to make sure the wound bed-wound agent interface is completely cleaned and closed with a bolstered dressing or vacuum-assisted closure. Patient education is essential to prevent shearing of the construct before ingrowth into the wound bed in places where these constructs are more challenging to hold [13].

Finally, seroma development is another regularly observed complication linked to the use of dermoconductive wound agents [87–90]. Given that thinner products are easier to incorporate than thicker ones and that seroma formation often results from extended engraftment, using thinner products may lower the likelihood of seroma formation [91].

7.2 Limitations

The effectiveness of biological wound treatments in specific clinical scenarios has been shown in numerous multicenter randomized controlled trials. Despite this, there is a lack of high-quality data for the off-label uses of many products, making it challenging for surgeons to explain their usefulness [78, 92]. Many biologic wound agents have a steep learning curve as compared to conventional skin grafting methods, which commonly causes new surgeons to have difficulties [19]. Lastly, there is little information available about how biologic wound agents affect the expenses associated with providing healthcare [93, 94]. Although these items are pricey, it is likely that, when compared to other reconstructive modalities, they will result in lower costs if they considerably cut the number of revisional surgeries needed after surgery. Furthermore, the use of biological wound agents has been severely constrained in low- and middle-income nations because of their expensive cost.

8. Conclusions

Through translational research, a better understanding of the physiology of wound healing has resulted in the creation of numerous biologic wound agents. Biologic wound agents have been successfully used in numerous therapeutic situations since they were originally used for burn surgery. While numerous studies including ones done at our institution have demonstrated the excellent efficacy of these products in reconstructing a variety of defects, many of their off-label applications have not undergone rigorous multi-institutional investigation. There is also little information contrasting dermoinductive and dermoconductive items. Moving forward, the authors anticipate that the refinement of present technologies, as well as the introduction of new products, will result in patients having better postoperative outcomes throughout time.

Conflict of interest

None to disclose.

Notes/thanks/other declarations.

Thank you to the UT Southwestern Department of Plastic Surgery for their support in providing facilities for our patients.

Author details

Monal Depani* and James F. Thornton*
Department of Plastic Surgery, University of Texas Southwestern, Dallas, TX, USA

*Address all correspondence to: monal.depani@utsouthwestern.edu
and james.thornton@utsouthwestern.edu

References

[1] Boer M, Duchnik E, Maleszka R, Marchlewicz M. Structural and biophysical characteristics of human skin in maintaining proper epidermal barrier function. Postepy Dermatologii Alergologii. 2016;**33**(1):1-5

[2] Romanovsky AA. Skin temperature: Its role in thermoregulation. Acta Physiologica (Oxford, England). 2014;**210**(3):498-507

[3] Janis JE, Kwon RK, Attinger CE. The new reconstructive ladder: Modifications to the traditional model. Plastic and Reconstructive Surgery. 2011;**127** (Suppl. 1):205S-212S

[4] Ozhathil DK, Tay MW, Wolf SE, Branski LK. A narrative review of the history of skin grafting in burn care. Medicina (Kaunas, Lithuania). 2021;**57**(4):380

[5] Zhang Z, Lv L, Mamat M, Chen Z, Liu L, Wang Z. Xenogenic (porcine) acellular dermal matrix is useful for the wound healing of severely damaged extremities. Experimental and Therapeutic Medicine. 2014;**7**(3):621-624

[6] Ferry AM, Beh HZ, Truong LA, et al. Management of bilateral temporomandibular joint ankylosis and class 2 malocclusion in a patient with Nager syndrome. FACE. 2021;**2**(04):484-489. DOI: 10.1177/27325016211055789

[7] Fosnot J, Kovach SJ III, Serletti JM. Acellular dermal matrix: General principles for the plastic surgeon. Aesthetic Surgery Journal. 2011;**31**(7):5S-12S

[8] Kim JJ, Evans GRD. Applications of biomaterials in plastic surgery. Clinics in Plastic Surgery. 2012;**39**(4):359-376

[9] Banyard DA, Bourgeois JM, Widgerow AD, Evans GRD. Regenerative biomaterials: A review. Plastic and Reconstructive Surgery. 2015;**135**(6):1740-1748

[10] Hughes OB, Rakosi A, Macquhae F, Herskovitz I, Fox JD, Kirsner RS. A review of cellular and acellular matrix products: Indications, techniques, and outcomes. Plastic and Reconstructive Surgery. 2016;**138**(3):138S-147S

[11] Protzman NM, Brigido SA. Recent advances in acellular regenerative tissue scaffolds. Clinics in Podiatric Medicine and Surgery. Jan 2015;**32**(1):147-159. DOI: 10.1016/j.cpm.2014.09.008. PMID: 25440425

[12] Novitsky YWMD, Rosen MJMD. The biology of biologics: Basic science and clinical concepts. Plastic and Reconstructive Surgery. 2012;**130**(5, Suppl 2):9S-17S

[13] Thornton JF, Carboy JA. Facial Reconstruction after Mohs Surgery. New York: Thieme Medical Publishers, Incorporated; 2018

[14] Gohari S, Gambla C, Healey M, et al. Evaluation of tissue-engineered skin (human skin substitute) and secondary intention healing in the treatment of full thickness wounds after Mohs micrographic or excisional surgery. Dermatologic Surgery. 2002;**28**(12):1107-1114. discussion 1114

[15] Gurtner GC, Garcia AD, Bakewell K, Alarcon JB. A retrospective matched-cohort study of 3994 lower extremity wounds of multiple etiologies across 644 institutions comparing a bioactive human skin allograft, TheraSkin, plus

standard of care, to standard of care alone. International Wound Journal. 2020;**17**(1):55-64

[16] Harding K, Sumner M, Cardinal M. A prospective, multicentre, randomised controlled study of human fibroblast-derived dermal substitute (Dermagraft) in patients with venous leg ulcers. International Wound Journal. 2013;**10**(2):132-137

[17] Tchanque-Fossuo CN, Dahle SE, Lev-Tov H, et al. Cellular versus acellular matrix devices in the treatment of diabetic foot ulcers: Interim results of a comparative efficacy randomized controlled trial. Journal of Tissue Engineering and Regenerative Medicine. 2019;**13**(8):1430-1437

[18] Lev-Tov H, Li CS, Dahle S, Isseroff RR. Cellular versus acellular matrix devices in treatment of diabetic foot ulcers: Study protocol for a comparative efficacy randomized controlled trial. Trials. 2013;**14**:18

[19] Vyas KS, Vasconez HC. Wound healing: Biologics, skin substitutes, biomembranes and scaffolds. Healthcare (Basel). 2014;**2**(3):356-400

[20] Veves A, Falanga V, Armstrong DG, Sabolinski ML, Apligraf Diabetic Foot Ulcer Study. Graftskin, a human skin equivalent, is effective in the management of noninfected neuropathic diabetic foot ulcers: A prospective randomized multicenter clinical trial. Diabetes Care. 2001;**24**(2):290-295

[21] Falanga V, Sabolinski M. A bilayered living skin construct (APLIGRAF) accelerates complete closure of hard-to-heal venous ulcers. Wound Repair and Regeneration. 1999;**7**(4):201-207

[22] Falanga V, Margolis D, Alvarez O, et al. Rapid healing of venous ulcers and lack of clinical rejection with an allogeneic cultured human skin equivalent. Human Skin Equivalent Investigators Group. Archives of Dermatology. 1998;**134**(3):293-300

[23] Marston WA, Hanft J, Norwood P, Pollak R, Dermagraft Diabetic Foot Ulcer Study Group. The efficacy and safety of Dermagraft in improving the healing of chronic diabetic foot ulcers: Results of a prospective randomized trial. Diabetes Care. 2003;**26**(6):1701-1705

[24] Frykberg RG, Marston WA, Cardinal M. The incidence of lower-extremity amputation and bone resection in diabetic foot ulcer patients treated with a human fibroblast-derived dermal substitute. Advances in Skin & Wound Care. 2015;**28**(1):17-20

[25] Zelen CM, Serena TE, Gould L, et al. Treatment of chronic diabetic lower extremity ulcers with advanced therapies: A prospective, randomised, controlled, multi-centre comparative study examining clinical efficacy and cost. International Wound Journal. 2016;**13**(2):272-282

[26] Serena TE, Carter MJ, Le LT SMJ, DT DM, EpiFix VLU study group. A multicenter, randomized, controlled clinical trial evaluating the use of dehydrated human amnion/chorion membrane allografts and multilayer compression therapy vs. multilayer compression therapy alone in the treatment of venous leg ulcers. Wound Repair and Regeneration. 2014;**22**(6):688-693

[27] Lavery LA, Fulmer J, Shebetka KA, et al. The efficacy and safety of Grafix(®) for the treatment of chronic diabetic foot ulcers: Results of a multi-centre, controlled, randomised, blinded, clinical trial. International Wound Journal. 2014;**11**(5):554-560

[28] Jeschke MG, Rose C, Angele P, Füchtmeier B, Nerlich MN, Bolder U. Development of new reconstructive techniques: Use of Integra in combination with fibrin glue and negative-pressure therapy for reconstruction of acute and chronic wounds. Plastic and Reconstructive Surgery. 2004;**113**(2):525-530

[29] Driver VR, Lavery LA, Reyzelman AM, et al. A clinical trial of Integra Template for diabetic foot ulcer treatment. Wound Repair and Regeneration. 2015;**23**(6):891-900

[30] Cazzell SM, Lange DL, Dickerson JE Jr, Slade HB. The management of diabetic foot ulcers with porcine small intestine submucosa tri-layer matrix: A randomized controlled trial. Advances in Wound Care (New Rochelle). 2015;**4**(12):711-718

[31] Mostow EN, Haraway GD, Dalsing M, Hodde JP, King D, OASIS Venus Ulcer Study Group. Effectiveness of an extracellular matrix graft (OASIS Wound Matrix) in the treatment of chronic leg ulcers: A randomized clinical trial. Journal of Vascular Surgery. 2005;**41**(5):837-843

[32] Kelechi TJ, Mueller M, Hankin CS, Bronstone A, Samies J, Bonham PA. A randomized, investigator-blinded, controlled pilot study to evaluate the safety and efficacy of a poly-N-acetyl glucosamine-derived membrane material in patients with venous leg ulcers. Journal of the American Academy of Dermatology. 2012;**66**(6):e209-e215

[33] Reynolds M, Kelly DA, Walker NJ, Crantford C, Defranzo AJ. Use of integra in the management of complex hand wounds from cancer resection and nonburn trauma. Hand (N. Y.). 2018;**13**(1):74-79

[34] Chavarriaga LF, Lin E, Losken A, et al. Management of complex abdominal wall defects using acellular porcine dermal collagen. The American Surgeon. 2010;**76**(1):96-100

[35] Wu-Fienberg Y, Wu SS, Gatherwright J, Chepla KJ. An alternative dermal template for reconstruction of complex upper extremity wounds. Plastic and Reconstructive Surgery. Global Open. 2021;**9**(7):e3674

[36] Hughes LP, Forman S, Krieg JC, Hughes WB. The use of integra dermal regeneration templates and cortical bone fenestrations over exposed tibia. Plastic and Reconstructive Surgery. Global Open. 2021;**9**(2):e3340

[37] Thornton JF, Griffin JR, Constantine FC. Nasal reconstruction: An overview and nuances. Seminars in Plastic Surgery. 2008;**22**(4):257-268

[38] Tiengo C, Amabile A, Azzena B. The contribution of a dermal substitute in the three-layers reconstruction of a nose tip avulsion. Journal of Plastic, Reconstructive & Aesthetic Surgery. 2012;**65**(1):114-117

[39] Seth AK, Ratanshi I, Dayan JH, Disa JJ, Mehrara BJ. Nasal reconstruction using the integra dermal regeneration template. Plastic and Reconstructive Surgery. 2019;**144**(4):966-970

[40] Gonyon DL Jr, Zenn MR. Simple approach to the radiated scalp wound using INTEGRA skin substitute. Annals of Plastic Surgery. 2003;**50**(3):315-320

[41] Harirah M, Sanniec K, Yates T, Harirah O, Thornton JF. Scalp reconstruction after Mohs cancer excision: Lessons learned from more than 900 consecutive cases. Plastic and Reconstructive Surgery. 2021;**147**(5):1165-1175

[42] Groeber F, Holeiter M, Hampel M, Hinderer S, Schenke-Layland K. Skin

tissue engineering–in vivo and in vitro applications. Advanced Drug Delivery Reviews. 2011;**63**(4-5):352-366

[43] Halim AS, Khoo TL, Mohd Yussof SJ. Biologic and synthetic skin substitutes: An overview. Indian Journal of Plastic Surgery. 2010;**43**(Suppl):S23-S28

[44] Parham MJ, Grush AE, Smerica A, Wen YE, Depani M, Ferry AM, Jones LM, Thornton JF. Overview of biologic agents used in skin and soft tissue reconstruction. InSeminars in Plastic Surgery. Thieme Medical Publishers, Inc; Feb 15 2022

[45] Bradford BD, Lee JW. Reconstruction of the forehead and scalp. Facial Plastic Surgery Clinics of North America. 2019;**27**(1):85-94

[46] Depani M, Grush AE, Parham MJ, Jones LM, Thornton JF. Use of biologic agents in nasal and scalp reconstruction. InSeminars in Plastic Surgery. Thieme Medical Publishers, Inc.; Mar 9 2022

[47] Rohrich RJ, Villanueva NL, Small KH, Pezeshk RA. Implications of facial asymmetry in rhinoplasty. Plastic and Reconstructive Surgery. 2017;**140**(3):510-516

[48] Cai LZ, Kwong JW, Azad AD, Kahn D, Lee GK, Nazerali RS. Where do we look? Assessing gaze patterns in cosmetic face-lift surgery with eye tracking technology. Plastic and Reconstructive Surgery. 2019;**144**(1):63-70

[49] Oneal RM, Beil RJ. Surgical anatomy of the nose. Clinics in Plastic Surgery. 2010;**37**(2):191-211

[50] Burget GC, Menick FJ. The subunit principle in nasal reconstruction. Plastic and Reconstructive Surgery. 1985;**76**(2):239-247

[51] Dey JK, Ishii LE, Byrne PJ, Boahene KDO, Ishii M. The social penalty of facial lesions: New evidence supporting high-quality reconstruction. JAMA Facial Plastic Surgery. 2015;**17**(2):90-96

[52] Baumann D, Robb G. Lip reconstruction. Seminars in Plastic Surgery. 2008;**22**(4):269-280

[53] Sarrami SM, Skochdopole AJ, Ferry AM, Buchanan EP, Hollier LH Jr, Dempsey RF. Revisional techniques for secondary cleft lip deformities. Seminars in Plastic Surgery. 2021;**35**(2):65-71

[54] Sanniec KJ, Carboy JA, Thornton JF. Simplifying lip reconstruction: An algorithmic approach. Seminars in Plastic Surgery. 2018;**32**(2):69-74

[55] Sanniec K, Harirah M, Thornton JF. Lip reconstruction after Mohs cancer excision: Lessons learned from 615 consecutive cases. Plastic and Reconstructive Surgery. 2020;**145**(2):533-542

[56] Chang SH, Huang ZS, Chen WL, Zhou B, Zhong JL. Vermilionectomy followed by reconstruction of the vermilion mucosa using allograft dermal matrix in patients with actinic cheilitis of the lower lip. Journal of Cosmetic Dermatology. 2021;**20**(1):263-266

[57] Pickert AJ, Nemeth Ochoa SA. Use of porcine xenografts on partial-thickness vermilion border and mucosal lower lip Mohs defects. Dermatologic Surgery. 2013;**39**(6):948-950

[58] Haslik W, Kamolz LP, Manna F, Hladik M, Rath T, Frey M. Management of full-thickness skin defects in the hand and wrist region: First long-term experiences with the dermal

matrix Matriderm. Journal of Plastic, Reconstructive & Aesthetic Surgery. 2010;**63**(2):360-364

[59] Meaike JD, Dickey RM, Killion E, Bartlett EL, Brown RH. Facial skin cancer reconstruction. Seminars in Plastic Surgery. 2016;**30**(3):108-121

[60] Rogers-Vizena CR, Lalonde DH, Menick FJ, Bentz ML. Surgical treatment and reconstruction of nonmelanoma facial skin cancers. Plastic and Reconstructive Surgery. 2015;**135**(5):895e-908e

[61] Heller L, Cole P, Kaufman Y. Cheek reconstruction: Current concepts in managing facial soft tissue loss. Seminars in Plastic Surgery. 2008;**22**(4):294-305

[62] Ebrahimi A, Ashayeri M, Rasouli HR. Comparison of local flaps and skin grafts to repair cheek skin defects. Journal of Cutaneous and Aesthetic Surgery. 2015;**8**(2):92-96

[63] Hamilton KL, Weathers WM, Wolfswinkel EM, Thornton JF. Repair of combined cheek and nose defects: Categorization and utilization. Seminars in Plastic Surgery. 2013;**27**(2):117-120

[64] Rapstine ED, Knaus WJ II, Thornton JF. Simplifying cheek reconstruction: A review of over 400 cases. Plastic and Reconstructive Surgery. 2012;**129**(6):1291-1299

[65] Nq Huynh M, Rokui S, McRae MC. An outcome comparison of superficial versus deep plane dissection of cervicofacial flaps: A systematic review and meta-analysis. Journal of Plastic, Reconstructive & Aesthetic Surgery. 2021;**74**(4):730-739

[66] Rogers HW, Weinstock MA, Feldman SR, Coldiron BM. Incidence estimate of nonmelanoma skin cancer (keratinocyte carcinomas) in the U.S. population, 2012. JAMA Dermatology. 2015;**151**(10):1081-1086

[67] Ferry AM, Sarrami SM, Hollier PC, Gerich CF, Thornton JF. Treatment of non-melanoma skin cancers in the absence of Mohs micrographic surgery. Plastic and Reconstructive Surgery. Global Open. 2020;**8**(12):e3300

[68] Hutchinson BL. Malignant melanoma in the lower extremity. A comprehensive overview. Clinics in Podiatric Medicine and Surgery. 1986;**3**(3):533-550

[69] Durbec F, Martin L, Derancourt C, Grange F. Melanoma of the hand and foot: Epidemiological, prognostic and genetic features. A systematic review. The British Journal of Dermatology. 2012;**166**(4):727-739

[70] Juzeniene A, Baturaite Z, Moan J. Sun exposure and melanomas on sun-shielded and sun-exposed body areas. Advances in Experimental Medicine and Biology. 2014;**810**:375-389

[71] Mun GH. Management of malignant melanoma. Archives of Plastic Surgery. 2012;**39**(5):565-574

[72] Bichakjian CK, Olencki T, Aasi SZ, et al. Basal cell skin cancer, version 1.2016, NCCN Clinical Practice Guidelines in Oncology. Journal of the National Comprehensive Cancer Network. 2016;**14**(5):574-597

[73] National Comprehensive Cancer Network Basal Cell and Squamous Cell Skin Cancers. Basal cell and squamous cell skin cancers. Clinical practice guidelines in oncology. Journal of the National Comprehensive Cancer Network. 2004;**2**(1):6-27

[74] Swetter SM, Tsao H, Bichakjian CK, et al. Guidelines of care for the management of primary cutaneous

melanoma. Journal of the American Academy of Dermatology. 2019;**80**(1):208-250

[75] Gimenez AR, Winocour SJ, Chu CK. Reconstructive techniques in melanoma for the surgical oncologist. Surgical Oncology Clinics of North America. 2020;**29**(3):349-367

[76] Shakir S, Messa CA IV, Broach RB, et al. Indications and limitations of bilayer wound matrix-based lower extremity reconstruction: A multidisciplinary case-control study of 191 wounds. Plastic and Reconstructive Surgery. 2020;**145**(3):813-822

[77] Cai A, Boos AM, Arkudas A, Horch RE. Management of extremely hard-to-heal extremity wounds with severe life-threatening complications. International Wound Journal. 2017;**14**(4):708-715

[78] Sarrami SM, Ferry AM, Buchanan EP, Gerow FT, Koshy JC. Reconstructing severe lower extremity skin necrosis in a pediatric patient. Advances in Skin & Wound Care. 2021;**34**(7):1-6

[79] Frame JD, Still J, Lakhel-LeCoadou A, et al. Use of dermal regeneration template in contracture release procedures: A multicenter evaluation. Plastic and Reconstructive Surgery. 2004;**113**(5):1330-1338

[80] Shores JT, Hiersche M, Gabriel A, Gupta S. Tendon coverage using an artificial skin substitute. Journal of Plastic, Reconstructive & Aesthetic Surgery. 2012;**65**(11):1544-1550

[81] Khundkar R. Lower extremity flap coverage following trauma. Journal of Clinical Orthopaedics and Trauma. 2019;**10**(5):839-844

[82] Hicks CW, Zhang GQ, Canner JK, et al. Outcomes and predictors of wound healing among patients with complex diabetic foot wounds treated with a dermal regeneration template (Integra). Plastic and Reconstructive Surgery. 2020;**146**(4):893-902

[83] Bebe FN, Hu S, Brown TL, Tulp OL. Role, extent, and impact of comorbidity on prognosis and survival in advanced metastatic melanoma: A review. The Journal of Clinical and Aesthetic Dermatology. 2019;**12**(1):16-23

[84] Han G, Ceilley R. Chronic wound healing: A Review of current management and treatments. Advances in Therapy. Mar 2017;**34**(3):599-610. DOI: 10.1007/s12325-017-0478-y. [Epub 2017 Jan 21]. PMID: 28108895; PMCID: PMC5350204

[85] Gonzalez SR, Wolter KG, Yuen JC. Infectious complications associated with the use of Integra: A systematic review of the literature. Plastic and Reconstructive Surgery. Global Open. 2020;**8**(7):e2869

[86] Chang DK, Louis MR, Gimenez A, Reece EM. The basics of integra dermal regeneration template and its expanding clinical applications. Seminars in Plastic Surgery. Aug 2019;**33**(3):185-189. DOI: 10.1055/s-0039-1693401. [Epub 2019 Aug 2]. PMID: 31384234; PMCID: PMC6680073

[87] Chun YS, Verma K, Rosen H, et al. Implant-based breast reconstruction using acellular dermal matrix and the risk of postoperative complications. Plastic and Reconstructive Surgery. 2010;**125**(2):429-436

[88] Chavarriaga LF, Lin E, Losken A, Cook MW, Jeansonne LO, White BC, et al. Management of complex abdominal wall defects using acellular porcine dermal collagen. The American Surgeon. Jan 2010;**76**(1):96-100. PMID: 20135948

[89] Brigido SA. The use of an acellular dermal regenerative tissue matrix in the treatment of lower extremity wounds: A prospective 16-week pilot study. International Wound Journal. 2006;**3**(3):181-187

[90] Shaikh FM, Giri SK, Durrani S, Waldron D, Grace PA. Experience with porcine acellular dermal collagen implant in one-stage tension-free reconstruction of acute and chronic abdominal wall defects. World Journal of Surgery. 2007;**31**(10):1966-1972. discussion 1973-1974, 1975

[91] Hur J, Han HH. Outcome assessment according to the thickness and direction of the acellular dermal matrix after implant-based breast reconstruction. BioMed Research International. 2021;**2021**:8101009

[92] Mustoe TA, Han H. The effect of new technologies on plastic surgery. Archives of Surgery. 1999;**134**(11):1178-1183

[93] Shahrokhi S, Arno A, Jeschke MG. The use of dermal substitutes in burn surgery: Acute phase. Wound Repair and Regeneration. 2014;**22**(1):14-22

[94] Sbitany H, Langstein HN. Acellular dermal matrix in primary breast reconstruction. Aesthetic Surgery Journal. 2011;**31**(7):30S-37S

Section 5

Treatment for Advanced Melanoma

Chapter 6

Immunotherapy of Metastatic Melanoma

Dan-Corneliu Jinga and Maria-Ruxandra Jinga

Abstract

Immunotherapy is part of the new treatments that significantly improved the prognostic of metastatic melanoma patients. The article reviews briefly the old immunotherapeutic approaches e.g., interferon-$\alpha 2$ and interleukin-2, and focuses on immune checkpoint inhibitors such as anti-CTLA-4 inhibitors and anti-PD-1 inhibitors in monotherapy or in combination (dual immune blockade). We detailed the results from CheckMate and KEYNOTTE clinical trials that lead to US Food and Drug Administration and European Medicines Agency approvals of the new agents for the treatment of advanced melanoma. The chapter concentrates on the algorithms for BRAF wild-type and BRAF mutated metastatic melanoma treatments, according to American (NCCN) and European (ESMO) guidelines. We underlined the first line, second line, and subsequent lines of treatment for both melanoma subtypes and for particular cases, such as in-transit metastasis or brain metastasis. A special attention was paid to treatment options for early and late disease progression (primary and acquired resistance after adjuvant therapy). Unfortunately, the new immune agents produce a higher toxicity rate, mainly immune adverse events. Also, these drugs can interact with the gut microbiome and with antibiotics, decreasing the efficacy of immune therapy. Finally, we review the new directions for immune therapy e.g., new immune combinations, the association of immune and targeted therapies, and adoptive cellular therapy with tumor-infiltrating lymphocytes, interleukin-2, and anti-PD-1.

Keywords: BRAF wild-type, BRAF mutated metastatic melanoma, immunotherapy, anti-CTLA-4, anti-PD-1, immune checkpoint inhibitors, dual immune blockade combination, immune-mediated adverse events, targeted therapy, primary resistance, acquired resistance, adoptive cellular therapy

1. Introduction

For more than a century, it is a known fact that cancer is an inflammatory disease and that immunotherapy (IT) can be used as a strategy for fighting it. Coley's toxin, utilized as early as 1893, can be considered the first IT approach in cancer [1].

At the beginning, the research was focused on the activation of the immune response using antitumor vaccines or direct stimulation with recombinant cytokines, e.g., interferons and interleukin-2 [2, 3].

Interferon alpha-2 (IFN-$\alpha 2$) was the first immunotherapeutic agent approved by the US Food and Drug Administration (FDA) in 1995, for adjuvant treatment of

IntechOpen

stages IIB-III melanoma patients, based on the results of the ECOG EST 1684 trial [4]. Previous outcomes of phase I/II studies demonstrated a tumor response rate of ~16%, but with a modest median duration of response (of ~4 months) for the treatment of disseminated melanoma [5, 6]. A meta-analysis of 13 trials published in 2018 showed a median relapse-free survival of 2.2 years (1.2–3.3 years) for the patients who received different IFN-α2b regimens, compared with 1.9 months for the patients that did not receive any adjuvant treatment for stages II and III [7].

The second cytokine approved by FDA in 1998 for the treatment of metastatic melanoma was Interleukin 2 (IL-2), due to its proven potential for durable disease control [8]. The administration of two cycles of high-dose IL-2 (HD-IL-2), each of them receiving 600,000 to 720,000 IU/Kg/per dose intravenously, every 8 hours, for up to a maximum of 14 doses per cycle, leads to clinical responses in ~16% of patients, including ~6% who had complete responses [9].

Unfortunately, the responses were infrequent and associated with severe side effects, especially for HD-IL-2, such as capillary leak syndrome (with hypotension, pulmonary edema, and renal failure), hepatic, gastrointestinal, endocrine, and cutaneous toxicities, arrhythmias, and psychiatric disturbances [10]. These toxicities generally resolve in a few days after stopping HD-IL-2 therapy, but the mortality rate related to this treatment is 1–2% [11].

The combination of cytokines, IFN-α and/or IL-2, with chemotherapeutic agents (e.g., cisplatin, vinblastine, and dacarbazine), also named bio-chemotherapy, can enhance the response rates, but at the cost of significantly increased toxicity. Multiple prospective randomized clinical trials failed to demonstrate significant improvement in survival compared to chemotherapy alone [12].

The understanding of the mechanisms through which the immune system fights against cancer represents one of the greatest breakthroughs in medicine over the last 15 years [13].

The interaction between Cytotoxic T Lymphocyte-associated antigen 4 (CTLA-4) and Programmed cell death 1 (PD-1) receptors and their ligands, discovered by the teams that won the 2018 Nobel Prize for Medicine, led by James Allison [14, 15] and Tasuku Honjo [16, 17], became the foundation of the development of immune checkpoint inhibitors (ICI).

Immune checkpoints (IC) are negative regulators of T-cell activation. Along with co-stimulatory molecules, they have an important role in maintaining self-tolerance.

2. CTLA-4 inhibitors

The anti-CTLA-4 monoclonal antibodies (mAbs) ipilimumab, a fully human IgG1, and tremelimumab, a fully human IgG2, were the first IC blocking drugs to enter clinical trials in oncology; however, the only one approved by FDA for metastatic melanoma was ipilimumab, in March 2011, initially as a single-therapy.

The approval of ipilimumab as monotherapy for unresectable stage III or stage IV melanoma was based on the results of two clinical trials, CA 184–002 [18] and CA 184–024 [19]. The first trial compared ipilimumab 3 mg/Kg, 4 cycles at 3-weeks interval, single-agent therapy or in combination with glycoprotein (gp-100) peptide vaccine, with gp-100 vaccine monotherapy [18]. The second trial compared ipilimumab 10 mg/Kg, 4 cycles at 3-weeks interval, in combination with dacarbazine, with dacarbazine alone until week 22; the responders (patients with stable disease or patients with an objective response, and no unresolved adverse events) received ipilimumab or placebo every 12 weeks thereafter as maintenance therapy [19]. The results of both trials showed, for the patients who received ipilimumab, an improved response rate and an increase in the duration of the response, in addition to better results for PFS (progression-free survival) and OS (overall survival) for both previously treated [18] or untreated advanced melanoma patients [19]. The CA 184–169 clinical trial compared the standard and high doses of ipilimumab; the survival results were not significantly different [20].

Pooled data from several phases II and phase III trials demonstrate a median survival time of 11.4 months for ipilimumab monotherapy [21]. The survival curves reached a plateau after 3 years and appeared stable even after 10 years [21]. In CA 184–024 trial, approximately 20% of the patients treated with ipilimumab showed longer overall survival compared with chemotherapy (18.2% 5-year OS for ipilimumab in combination with dacarbazine versus 8.8% for dacarbazine alone) [22].

The real-world data from the Expanded Access Program for Ipilimumab confirmed the efficacity of this therapy for previously treated metastatic melanoma patients [23–30]. More than 1600 patients were treated with single-agent ipilimumab 3 mg/Kg, 4 cycles at 3-weeks interval (induction phase). The median PFS and median OS were similar between 6 European countries and South Africa (**Table 1**).

Safety results showed a high risk, 10–15%, of severe (grade 3 and 4) immune-mediated adverse events (irAEs) for standard dose ipilimumab monotherapy [18], 30% for high-dose ipilimumab monotherapy [20], and 38% risk of severe irAEs for ipilimumab combined with dacarbazine [19]. The study CA 184–002 reported seven deaths caused by immune-mediated AEs [18].

As a result, clinical guidelines do not recommend the association of ipilimumab with dacarbazine due to high risk for severe adverse events, and the FDA-recommended dose of ipilimumab is now 3 mg/Kg instead of 10 mg/Kg, 4 cycles at 3-weeks interval (induction therapy) [31].

The second anti-CTLA-4 antibody, tremelimumab, also generated promising anticancer responses in early clinical trials [32]. Unfortunately, a phase III clinical trial of tremelimumab versus standard-of-care chemotherapy in advanced melanoma was stopped early due to a lack of survival benefits [33].

Country	Patients number	median PFS (months)	median OS (months)	1-year OS (%)	2-year OS (%)
Czech Republic (23)	196	—	7.5	—	—
Italy (24)	855	3.7	7.2	—	—
Netherlands (25)	31	—	7	45.2	28.8
Poland (26)	50	3	8	—	—
Romania (27)	89	4.13	6.3	—	—
Spain (28)	144	—	6.5	32.9	—
South Africa (29)	108	3.44	—	36	20
UK (30)	193	2.8	6.1	31	14.8
Total	**1616**	**(2.8–4.13)**	**(6.1–8)**	**(31–45.2%)**	**14.8–28.8%**

Table 1.
The efficacity of ipilimumab monotherapy; results from expanded access program in 6 European countries and South-Africa (23–30).

3. PD-1 inhibitors

The anti-PD-1 monoclonal antibodies, pembrolizumab, and nivolumab, humanized immunoglobulins (IgG4), were both approved as single-agent therapies by FDA in 2014 for unresectable advanced or metastatic melanoma.

Pembrolizumab is administered intravenously at 2 mg/Kg body weight, or 200 mg fixed dose every 3 weeks until progression of the disease or until a severe toxicity develops. The treatment can be administered continuously, over a period of 1–2 years, depending on the response of the disease and the tolerance of the treatment. However, the optimal treatment duration has not been established until now [34].

The initial results from the phase I KEYNOTE-001 clinical trial showed a response rate of 34% and a median OS of 25.9 months for ipilimumab refractory metastatic melanoma [35]. The KEYNOTE-002 clinical trial compared two pembrolizumab doses (2 mg/Kg and 10 mg/Kg every 3 weeks) with chemotherapy for the same population as the previous study [36]. Long-term follow-up showed that both doses of pembrolizumab provide higher response rates (22–28%) and longer duration of response along with improvements in progression-free survival (16–22% PFS 2-year rate), compared with chemotherapy (4% response rate and < 1% PFS 2-year rate) [37]. Furthermore, pembrolizumab therapy was better tolerated than chemotherapy [38].

In the end, the results of phase III KEYNOTE-006 clinical trial support the recommendation of American (NCCN) and European (ESMO) guidelines that pembrolizumab should be considered as first-line therapy in patients with unresectable or metastatic melanoma [39, 40]. The clinical trial compared two pembrolizumab regimens (10 mg/Kg every 2 or every 3 weeks) with ipilimumab for the patients with metastatic melanoma previously untreated with ICI [41, 42]. All the study endpoints aligned: 36–37% response rate for pembrolizumab compared with 13% for ipilimumab (statistically significant), 28–31% PFS 2-year rate versus 14% for ipilimumab (statistically significant), and a trend to improve the OS 2-year rate for pembrolizumab [42].

The kinetics of the response to pembrolizumab reflects the response to immunotherapy. Long-term follow-up during clinical trials showed a late response to pembrolizumab therapy, more than a year after the start of the treatment; in addition, some partial responders may become complete responders over time [37, 41, 43].

Nivolumab is administered intravenously at 3 mg/Kg body weight or 240 mg fixed dose every 2 weeks, or 480 mg fixed dose every 4 weeks until progression of the disease or until a severe toxicity develops.

The phase III study CheckMate 037 compared nivolumab with chemotherapy for the patients with ipilimumab-refractory metastatic melanoma (BRAF wild-type) and for the patients with ipilimumab and BRAF inhibitors refractory metastatic melanoma (BRAF mutated) [44]. Immunotherapy improved the response rate (27% versus 10%) and the duration of the response compared with chemotherapy, but after 2 years, it did not improve neither median PFS (3.1 versus 3.7 months) nor median OS (15.7 versus 14.7 months) [44, 45].

The subsequent phase III CheckMate 066 and 067 clinical trials demonstrated nivolumab efficacy in unresectable stage III and metastatic stage IV melanoma. In CheckMate 066, nivolumab monotherapy was compared with chemotherapy [46, 47]. The response rate (40% versus 13.9%), median PFS (5.1 versus 2.2 months), and median OS (37.5 versus 11.2 months) were statistically significant in favor of immunotherapy [46, 47]. Nivolumab therapy led to long-term survival in up to 40% of patients, as the survival curves suggest [47].

In the CheckMate 067 clinical trial, the dual immune combination of CTLA-4 and PD-1 inhibitors was compared with nivolumab (monotherapy) and with ipilimumab (monotherapy) as first-line treatments for metastatic melanoma; the results demonstrated the superiority of dual immune combination and also of single-agent PD-1 inhibitor over ipilimumab monotherapy [48–50]. In monotherapy, nivolumab was superior to ipilimumab in terms of response rate (45% versus 19%), median PFS (6.9 versus 2.9 months), and median OS (36.9 versus 19.9 months) [48–50].

The kinetics of the response to nivolumab, ipilimumab, and pembrolizumab was almost identical, with late complete response seen more than a year after the start of the treatment [45, 48, 50]. Across clinical trials, response to nivolumab tends to persist after the discontinuation of the drug [48, 50].

4. Dual immune blockade (CTLA-4 and PD-1 Inhibitors)

Preclinical studies demonstrated that dual immune blockade with anti-CTLA-4 combined with anti-PD-1 was more effective than with either alone [51]. A phase I study of immune combination therapies found that the maximum tolerated dose of concurrent administration is 3 mg/Kg q3w for ipilimumab and 1 mg/Kg for nivolumab q3w; in this study, the overall response rate was 40% and the grade 3–4 AEs rate was 53% [52].

The nivolumab and ipilimumab combination arms from CheckMate 067 and CheckMate 069 clinical trials showed higher response rates (58% vs. 19%, $p < 0.001$ for CheckMate 067 and 59% vs. 11% for CheckMate 069), prolonged response durations, longer time to subsequent therapies, prolonged median PFS (11.5 vs. 2.9 months, $p < 0.001$ for CheckMate 067 and not reached vs. 3.0 months in CheckMate 069), and larger median OS compared with single-agent ipilimumab [50, 53]. These effects persisted during long-term follow-up, with 4-year survival rates of 53% for the combination arm compared with 46% for single-agent nivolumab and with 30% for single-agent ipilimumab in the CheckMate 067 study [48]. For a subgroup of patients with high levels of PD-L1 expression, the median OS and median PFS were similar for single-agent nivolumab compared with the ipilimumab and nivolumab combination, but the number of toxicities was smaller for monotherapy [48].

Long-term follow-up (6.5 years) in the CheckMate 067 study showed a longer median OS of 72.1, 36.9, and 19.9 months in the combination arm compared with nivolumab and ipilimumab monotherapy [54].

CheckMate 067 and 069 showed significantly increased toxicity of dual immune blockade versus monotherapy [50, 53]. The rate of grade 3–4 related adverse events (AEs) in CheckMate 067 was 59% for the ipilimumab and nivolumab arm compared with 21% for nivolumab alone and with 28% for ipilimumab monotherapy [50]. In CheckMate 069 the rate of AEs for the combination was 54%, compared with 20% for ipilimumab monotherapy [53].

A pooled analysis of the immune combination trials found that response rates, PFS, and OS of the patients who discontinued the treatment in the induction phase due to the AE, were similar to those of the patients who completed the treatment [55].

The kinetics of the response to combination therapy includes a late complete response (CR) that was seen more than a year after the start of treatment, with a double rate of CR, and increased response duration [48, 49].

Subgroup analysis, in both CheckMate clinical studies, demonstrated improved efficacy with nivolumab and ipilimumab combination therapy, regardless of BRAF mutation status [48–50, 53].

In order to identify a possible biomarker that could predict the response to immunotherapy, the researchers assessed PD-L1 expression in tumor samples from the patients included in CheckMate and KEYNOTE trials [45, 47–50, 56]. In these randomized clinical studies, the improved response rate, PFS, and OS for anti-PD-1 therapy had a statistically significant correlation with increased PD-L1 expression, [45, 46, 48–50, 56].

However, it was not possible to identify an expression level cutoff for PD-L1 with a cert prognostic value. Furthermore, in these clinical trials, there were patients who experienced durable responses to anti-PD-1 inhibitors, regardless of the PD-L1 expression in biopsy specimens [56].

At the present time, we know the following [39]:

1. Anti-PD-1 therapy (nivolumab) and dual immune therapy (ipilimumab in combination with nivolumab) efficacies appear to improve with increasing PD-L1 expression; however, this biomarker is not the only one that predicts the response to ICI [48].

2. For high PD-L1 tumor expression, improvements in outcome with dual immune therapy or with nivolumab monotherapy were similar; instead, for low PD-L1 tumor expression, the outcome was better with dual immune therapy [48].

3. Unlike CTLA-4 inhibitor monotherapy, the dual immune therapy led to good responses even in patients with very low PD-L1 tumor expression [48].

4. PD-L1 tumor expression cannot be used in order to exclude patients from anti-PD-1 monotherapy [39]; however, the use of combination therapy for patients with low PD-L1 tumor expression, in order to increase efficacy, and the use of PD-L1 monotherapy for patients with a high level of PD-L1 tumor expression, in order to decrease the toxicity, prove effective and are consequently preferred [39].

Treatment for stage III In-transit melanoma represents a real challenge for medical oncologists, dermatologists, and surgeons. Local therapy (e.g., intralesional injections) can be combined with regional therapy (e.g., Isolated Limb Perfusion and Infusion) and systemic therapy [39].

Talimogen laherparepvec (T-VEC), an agent that uses a modified herpes simplex virus to induce tumor cell lysis and deliver a localized expression of GM-CSF is the main intralesional agent approved for this indication, according to the results of a phase 3 clinical study [57]. T-VEC produced local durable response rates (16.3% versus 2.1% for injection of GM-CSF) and remission of oligometastatic disease (bystander effect). The overall response rate was superior for intralesional T-VEC compared with intralesional GM-CSF (26.4% vs. 5.7%, $p < 0.001$) with higher rates of complete response (11% vs. 1%) [57].

The AEs rate produced by T-VEC injection was 20%, with 11% serious-AEs (grade 3–4). The most frequent AEs were local, e.g., injection-site reactions (cellulitis, pain, and peripheral edema), but also systemic toxicities appeared (fatigue, chills, pyrexia, and other flu-like symptoms) [57].

Immune Checkpoint Inhibitors combined with T-VEC intralesional injections represent a new approach in clinical ongoing trials. At first, the combination ipilimumab with T-VEC was tested, with a spectacular reduction of tumor burden for the injected lesions and also for some distant lesions [58]. However, the good clinical response did not engender longer PFS, and the rate of AEs was higher for the combination, compared with both agents in monotherapy. The phase 3 MASTERKEY-265 trial combined pembrolizumab with T-VEC in order to improve previous results by reducing toxicities [59]. The anti-PD-1 and T-VEC combination demonstrated a 43% CR with 4-year PFS and OS rates of 55.9 and 71.4%, respectively [59].

5. Immune Checkpoint Inhibitors (ICI) and Brain Metastasis (BM)

Treatment of melanoma BM is a real challenge for oncologists and radiotherapists. Clinical studies confirmed that immune therapy can be used safely and efficiently, especially in asymptomatic patients with BM. The CA 184–042 study demonstrates the superiority of HD-ipilimumab in asymptomatic patients (compared with symptomatic patients) in terms of response rate (16% vs. 5%), median PFS (2.6 vs. 1.3 months), and median OS (7.0 months vs. 3.7 months). Interestingly, good response rates were obtained for both intracranial and extracranial disease [60]. The patients with asymptomatic BM from the CA 184–169 trial had the same median OS for HD-ipilimumab and for standard ipilimumab doses [20].

For PD-1 inhibitors, used in the asymptomatic BM population, clinical studies showed good response rates, 30% for pembrolizumab [61] and 29% for nivolumab [62], and also high median OS (17 months for pembrolizumab and 18.5 months for nivolumab) [61, 62]. In the subset of patients with symptomatic BM and leptomeningeal disease, usually with bad prognostic, the CA 209–170 study finds a comparable response rate (25%), to the response rate (29%) for asymptomatic BM, but with much lower median OS (5.1 vs. 18. months) [62].

The real impact on asymptomatic BM patients was seen in the CA 209–170 clinical trial arm treated with a dual combination of ipilimumab and nivolumab, with 57% response rate for extracranial disease and 46% for intracranial disease; the median OS was not reached for immune combination, compared with 18.5 months for nivolumab monotherapy [62]. The good results for dual combination were confirmed by the CheckMate 204 clinical trial, with a more than 50% response rate for both extra and intracranial disease and with median OS not reached [63].

NCCN and ESMO guidelines concluded that ipilimumab and nivolumab combination is superior to anti-PD-1 monotherapy and that anti-PD-1 therapy provides higher response rates and better median OS compared with ipilimumab monotherapy, especially for asymptomatic BM melanoma patients [39, 40].

Accordingly, whole-brain radiotherapy (WBRT) is now reserved, only with palliative intent, for symptomatic BM patients [40]. Stereotactic radiosurgery (SRS) has replaced WBRT for non-bulky (< 3 cm), <5–10 asymptomatic BM, as upfront therapy. For more advanced disease, guidelines recommend first-line systemic therapy, mainly combination immune therapy; in this case, SRS will be used as salvage therapy for disease progression [40]. SRS and immune therapy can be administered simultaneously, but with close MRI evaluation, as a result of the increased risk for asymptomatic radio-necrosis (15% of patients) [64].

6. The algorithm for BRAF wild-type (wt) melanoma treatment

The current first-line standard therapies for inoperable stage III and IV BRAF wt melanoma are the PD-1 blockade (nivolumab or pembrolizumab) and the dual blockade CTLA-4 and PD-1 (ipilimumab and nivolumab) (**Table 2**) [39, 40]. Different regimens and doses from clinical guidelines are underlined in **Table 3**.

T-VEC is also an option for in-transit unresectable melanoma.

For second-line treatment and beyond, ESMO guidelines [40] recommend clinical trials if available, or ICI rechallenge.

Immune therapy rechallenge includes at least 3 options [40]:

- Ipilimumab after PD-1 monotherapy (nivolumab or pembrolizumab) [65]
- Nivolumab or pembrolizumab if another line of treatment was given after ICI failure (e.g., chemotherapy)
- Ipilimumab and nivolumab combination if not given previously [66]

Two clinical trials demonstrated that immune therapy with ipilimumab or with the dual combination ipilimumab and anti-PD-1 should be considered a viable

Inoperable stage III/IV melanoma		
	Therapy	**Melanoma subtype**
First-line	Immune therapy • Anti-PD-1/Anti-CTLA-4 combination • Anti-PD-1 monotherapy • T-VEC	BRAF wt BRAF mutated
	Targeted therapy BRAFi + MEKi	BRAF mutated
Second-line	Clinical Trial (after IT)	BRAF wt
	IT rechallenge: • ipilimumab after PD-1 monotherapy • PD-1 therapy after bridging treatment (e.g., chemo) • anti-PD-1 and anti-CTLA-4 combination if it is not given previously	BRAF wt
	Switched therapy (TT after IT or IT after TT)	BRAF mutated
Subsequent lines	• pembrolizumab / low dose ipilimumab combination for tumors that have progressed after prior anti-PD-1 therapy • HD-IL-2* • Ipilimumab and intralesional T-VEC combination* • pembrolizumab and Lenvatinib combination* • BSC	BRAF wt
	• rechallenge with both TT and IT • chemotherapy** • BSC	BRAF mutated

**Only for NCCN guideline [39].*
***Only for ESMO guideline [40].*

Table 2.
Algorithm for inoperable stage III/IV melanoma treatment (IT – Immune therapy; TT – Targeted therapy; BSC – Best supportive care).

Treatment	Dosing	Treatment duration
Nivolumab	240 mg q2w or 480 mg q4w	• until disease progression or unacceptable toxicity; • most common regimens in daily-practice
	3 mg/Kg q2w	• until disease progression or unacceptable toxicity; • it is allowed to continue the treatment for clinical benefit even in the case of progression of disease.
Pembrolizumab	200 mg q3w	• until disease progression or unacceptable toxicity; • most common regimens in daily-practice
	2 mg/Kg q3w 10 mg/Kg q2w or q3w	• until disease progression or unacceptable toxicity; • the treatment can be stopped after 24 months for complete responders
Ipilimumab / Nivolumab combination	1 mg/Kg nivo + 3 mg/kgc ipi q3w for 4 doses, followed by nivo 240 mg q2w or 480 mg q4w	• until disease progression or unacceptable toxicity;
	1 mg/kg nivo + 3 mg/kgc ipi q3w for 4 doses, followed by 3 mg/kg nivo monotherapy q2w	• until disease progression or unacceptable toxicity; • it is allowed to continue the treatment for clinical benefit even in the case of progression of disease.

Adapted from NCCN guideline [40].

Table 3.
Immune checkpoint inhibitor treatment regimens.

treatment option after failure of anterior PD-1 therapy [65, 66]. The combination appeared to be highly effective in terms of response rate, duration of the response, and median OS compared with ipilimumab monotherapy (20.4 vs. 8.8 months for median OS) [66]. The grade 3–5 toxicities for both groups were the same [66].

The NCCN guidelines have additional recommendations [39]:

- Pembrolizumab + low-dose ipilimumab combination for tumors that progressed after prior anti-PD-1 therapy [66]
- HD-IL-2
- Ipilimumab + intralesional T-VEC combination
- Pembrolizumab + lenvatinib combination

The combination of anti-PD-1 (pembrolizumab) with VEGF inhibitor (lenvatinib) produces a higher overall response rate of 48% compared with pembrolizumab alone, in a small phase I/II trial [67].

In particular cases, other options can be considered, such as imatinib for tumors with activating mutations of Kit, larotrectinib, and entrectinib for NTRK gene fusion-positive tumors [68] and cytotoxic agents.

7. The algorithm for BRAF mutated melanoma treatment

The current first-line treatment for inoperable stage III and IV BRAF-mutated melanoma is also immune therapy (IT), or the dual combination of BRAF inhibitors with MEK inhibitors (TT, Targeted Therapy) (**Table 2**). The best sequence of IT and TT is currently unknown [69]. No direct randomized comparison exists between IT and TT, but one meta-analysis suggests a better outcome after 1 year in favor of IT [70, 71], despite a very good response rate to TT in the first 12 months [72]. The main advantage of immune therapy as a first option is long-term/durable disease control even after treatment is ended [73].

There are several ongoing trials that study the optimal sequence for the first-line treatment, TT-IT or IT-TT (SECOMBIT, DREAMseq). Randomized three-arm phase 2 study (SECOMBIT / NCT02631447) revealed a better trend for OS and total PFS at 2 and 3 years for the arm with upfront ipilimumab and nivolumab combination and for the arm with short targeted therapy followed by immune combination therapy, compared with upfront targeted therapy with BRAFi + MEKi [74]. A randomized DREAMseq trial was designed to compare the efficacy and toxicity of the sequence IT-TT (Ipilimumab + nivolumab – dabrafenib + trametinib) with the sequence TT-IT. OS and duration of overall response (DOR) were better for upfront immune combination therapy (2-year OS of 72% vs. 52% $p = 0.0095$ and median DOR not reached for upfront immune therapy, and 12.7 months for targeted therapy) [75].

ESMO recommendation [76]:

- Elevated LDH level: ipilimumab and nivolumab combination preferred.
- LDH >1x and ≤ 2x ULN – anti-PD-1 monotherapy preferred.
- The tumor burden is not clearly defined yet.
- Switching TT to IT after short therapy should not be considered outside clinical trials.

First-line therapy selection for BRAF-mutated melanoma should be based on treatment goals (short-term benefit or long-term benefit), on the clinical characteristics of the disease (LDH level, organs involved, number of metastases or tumor burden, disease progression kinetics), on co-morbidities and performance status of the patient, and on the patient's preference and compliance for oral or iv agents [76]. However, it seems prudent to start with immune therapy for the cases with tumors that do not progress very quickly and do not immediately threaten an important organ or function [40].

ESMO recommendation [76]:

- Patients treated by TT-IT sequence can be rechallenged with targeted therapy.
- Patients treated by IT-TT sequence can be rechallenged with anti-PD-1 therapy (no data exist for ipilimumab and nivolumab combination).
- Patients treated with first-line anti-PD1 monotherapy and second-line TT might benefit from ipilimumab-based treatment.

- Finally, after using all options, rechallenge with the drugs that showed the best response should be considered.

As a second-line treatment, NCCN and ESMO guidelines recommend the switch from one treatment to another, depending on the previously used first-line therapy (**Table 2**) [39, 40].

Subsequent lines are not well established; as an option, clinical trials or rechallenge with both TT and IT can be considered. Another option can be chemotherapy with single-agent DTIC or Temozolomide, and Paclitaxel + Carboplatin combination, with palliative intent or as "bridging therapy" (**Table 2**).

8. Stopping immunotherapy in metastatic melanoma treatment

ESMO recommendation [76]:

- Stopping anti-PD-1 therapy for patients with CR that persist on radiological evaluation and who received treatment for at least 6 months should be considered.

- Stopping anti-PD-1 therapy for patients with PR and SD after 2 years of treatment should be considered.

- Stopping targeted therapy outside clinical trials is not recommended.

Sixty-seven patients from KEYNOTE-001 trial stopped the pembrolizumab therapy after complete response (CR) was confirmed by radiological evaluation and after completing minimum 6 months of treatment [43]. The 2-years DFS from the time of CR was ~90% [43]. In KEYNOTE-006 the patients stopped the treatment after 2 years and 85.4% did not suffer a relapse after 5 years of follow-up [77].

Both CheckMate 067 and KEYNOTE-006 trials revealed a good Hazard Ratio (HR) for progressive disease (PD) after 2 years with anti-PD-1 monotherapy (nivolumab, respectively pembrolizumab) for responders (partial response – PR and stable disease – SD) [43, 48].

9. Treatment for patients with disease progression after adjuvant therapy

ESMO recommendation [76]:

- The patients with primary resistance should be treated with another option.

- The patients with acquired resistance can be treated with the same treatment option or with another agent.

- The decision should be taken in accordance with BRAF status

Primary resistance (disease progression during the 12-months adjuvant therapy or < 6 months from the treatment ending): it is unlikely to have a clinical benefit from using the same agent [76, 78].

Acquired resistance (disease progression >6 months from the treatment ending): it is possible to use the same agent or an alternative agent from the same class [76, 79].

A multicenter randomized clinical study with 300 metastatic melanoma patients (56% BRAF wt and 44% BRAF mutated) evaluated the treatment for the patients who stopped responding after the initial response (acquired resistance) [78]. The most commonly used agent after the first progression was anti-PD-1 (51% of patients from the cohort study), followed by targeted therapy (19%), dual immune combination CTLA-4 and PD-1 (12%), investigational drugs (11%), and ipilimumab monotherapy (6%). The ORR was 46% for anti-PD-1 monotherapy, 67% for TT, 56% for immune combination therapy, 20% for the investigational agent, and 0% for CTLA-4 monotherapy, but no difference in OS after about 2 years of follow up was observed [78]. Another clinical trial demonstrated a higher response rate for the patients treated with the immune dual combination, compared with ipilimumab monotherapy for patients with progressive metastatic melanoma after first-line anti-PD-1 therapy (31% vs. 13%) [66].

A multicenter randomized clinical trial, that focused on the treatment of recurrence after adjuvant therapy, demonstrated a very good response to immune checkpoint inhibitors, similar to the response rate for the patients treated by first-line immune therapy; the three-year OS was 79% for anti-PD-1 based therapy (monotherapy or dual immune combination), 55% for targeted therapy rechallenge, and 25% for ipilimumab monotherapy [80].

10. Immune adverse events iAEs

The current treatments for melanoma produce high-grade toxicity rates, with 55–59% for ipilimumab and nivolumab combination, 20% for nivolumab alone, and 27% for ipilimumab alone [78]. The most common AEs associated with immune checkpoint inhibitors are autoimmune (iAEs). The most frequent immune toxicities to ICI, across all options (anti-PD-1 monotherapy, anti-CTLA-4 monotherapy, or dual immune combination), were cutaneous (pruritus, maculopapular rash, and vitiligo), gastrointestinal (diarrhea/colitis) and fatigue [39]. The most common high-grade, potentially life-threatening iAEs were endocrinopathies (hypophysitis, adrenal insufficiency, and hypo- or hyperthyroidism), pancreatitis, and hepatic AEs (elevated ALT, AST, hepatitis) [39]. Other potentially lethal iAEs were nephritis, pneumonitis, and myocarditis.

A retrospective study from the WHO pharmacovigilance database identified 613 fatal ICI toxic events, reported from 2009 to 2018. The most death-related AEs were pneumonitis, hepatitis, and neurotoxic effects, for the dual immune combination and colitis for anti-CTLA-4 treatment [81]. A meta-analysis of 112 trials showed higher toxicity-related fatality rates for CTLA-4 and PD-1 combination (1.23%) and for anti-CTLA-4 monotherapy (1.08%), compared with single-agent anti-PD-1 (0.36%) [81].

The treatment with ICI requires a routine monitoring for immune toxicities, with physical examination, anamnesis for autoimmune or infectious diseases (screening for HIV, hepatitis A, B, and C), complete blood count, comprehensive metabolic panel, cardiac evaluation with ECG and measurements of oxygen saturation, and endocrine evaluation (TSH, FT4 and serum cortisone), at baseline and periodically, for the entire treatment duration [82]. The NCCN elaborated a comprehensive guideline for the management of immunotherapy-related toxicities [82].

The kinetics of iAEs is different for different types of immune-related toxicities. The first toxicities that become evident are skin-related AEs (median time to onset 3 weeks), but the risk persists throughout treatment. Later, gastrointestinal (median time to onset 7 weeks) and hepatic toxicities appear, and finally pulmonary, endocrine, and renal AEs may develop [83, 84]. The patients who experienced AEs of any grade had a significantly higher objective response rate [83]. Most treatment-related AEs resolve completely after specific treatment, with the exception of endocrinopathies, which require long-term hormone replacement therapy [84]. Median time to resolution for grade 3–4 iAEs was under 5 weeks, apart from endocrinopathies excepted [84].

11. Immune checkpoint inhibitors and their impact on intestinal flora

ESMO recommendation [76]:

- Restrictive use of empirical antibiotics in melanoma patients treated by immune checkpoint inhibitors

Specific species of gut microbiome or microbiota can influence antitumoral responses, either through innate or adaptive immune pathways. In severely immunocompromised patients, the modification of intestinal flora through diet or fecal microbiota transplants could improve the response to ICI [85].

On the other hand, the excessive use of antibiotics decreases the diversity of gut microbiome and eliminates the most immunogenic bacteria, having thus a negative impact on patients treated with ICI [86].

12. New directions for immune therapy

12.1 Anti-LAG-3 and Anti-PD-1 immune combination

Lymphocyte-activation gene 3 (LAG-3) is a cell-surface receptor on activated CD4+ T cells and represents an alternate immune checkpoint [87]. The anti-LAG-3 agent relatlimab and anti-PD-1 agent nivolumab were combined in phase II/III RELATIVITY-047 clinical study [88]. The study compared the dual immune combination relatlimab and nivolumab with nivolumab monotherapy, favoring the immune combination in terms of median PFS (10.1 months for combination vs. 4.6 months for monotherapy, with HR for progression or death of 0.75). The obtained results were better for a subgroup of patients with positive LAG-3 expression ($\geq$ 1%). The rate of AEs was 18.9% for the combination and 9.7% for the monotherapy group [88].

In the CheckMate 067 clinical trial, PFS for the nivolumab and ipilimumab combination, the current first-line indication for stage III and IV inoperable melanoma, was 11.5 months, with a 59% rate of AEs [48]. If the first results of the RELATIVITY-047 clinical study will be supported also by better overall survival rates, it would give good grounds for the expectation that the relatlimab and nivolumab combination will replace the ipilimumab and nivolumab combination in the first-line treatment of metastatic melanoma [89].

12.2 Other Novel ICIs

Anti-VISTA small molecule ICI (CA 170) combined with nivolumab and anti-Tim-3 antibody combined with spartalizumab (anti-PD-1) are among the most promising immune combinations for the treatment of advanced melanoma [90, 91]. V-domain immunoglobulin suppressor of T-cell activation (VISTA) is a negative regulator of T-cell function; anti-VISTA agents show synergistic effects with anti-PD-1 agents [90]. T-cell immunoglobulin and mucin domain 3 (Tim-3) is a cell surface molecule expressed on lymphocytes, dendritic cells, and tumor cells (including melanoma cells) that breaks off T-cell activation and diminishes antitumor immunity [91]. Anti-Tim-3 monoclonal antibody stops T-cell inhibition and amplifies tumor cell disintegration.

Other potential new immune combinations are the associations between anti-PD-1 inhibitors with agonists of IL-2 described in the PIVOT-02 phase II clinical trial [92], or between anti-PD-1 agents and different oncolytic viruses (e.g., polio, coxsackie, herpes simplex or poxvirus) [93].

12.3 Adoptive cellular therapy (ACT)

ACT with the use of tumor-infiltrating lymphocytes (TILs) can be a future option for solid tumors, including metastatic melanoma [69, 94]. The clinical development of TILs started more than 40 years ago, but it was not approved by FDA for melanoma treatment, despite the good response rates [93]. The combination of TILs with chemotherapy and IL-2 was associated with a 24% CR and with 55% ORR among patients with disease recurrence after previous systemic treatment [94]. Because of high rates of potentially lethal AEs, this therapy can be safely administered only in a high-facility oncological center, trained for IL-2 administration.

One of the pivotal multicenter clinical trials was designed to evaluate TILs administration (lifileucel, an autologous, centrally manufactured TILs) in conjunction with IL-2, followed by sequential ICI, in patients with solid tumors, including melanoma (NCT 02360579) [95]. The ORR was 36%, with 2 from 66 patients with CR and 22 from 66 patients with PR. Median duration of response was not reached after 18.7 months of median follow-up. This treatment could be used as salvage therapy for metastatic melanoma patients, refractory to anti-PD-1 and targeted therapy [95].

Systemic treatment for metastatic melanoma improved dramatically in the last 10 years with enhanced long-term survival of these patients. Immune therapy is part of the change of the treatment paradigm in melanoma; shifting from direct cytotoxic tumor destruction to increasing the immune system activity in order to destroy the cancer cells. Undoubtedly, the near future will be the time of different dual immune combinations, with or without new targeted therapy approaches.

Author details

Dan-Corneliu Jinga[1]* and Maria-Ruxandra Jinga[2]

1 Department of Medical Oncology and Hematology, Neolife Bucharest Medical Center, Romania

2 Medical School, Newcastle University, United Kingdom

*Address all correspondence to: danjinga2002@yahoo.com

References

[1] Coley WB. The treatment of malignant tumors by repeated inoculations of erysipelas. With a report of ten original cases. Clinical Orthopaedics and Related Research. 1991;**262**:3-11

[2] Harris SJ, Brown J, Lopez J, Yap TA. Immuno-oncology combinations: Raising the tail of the survival curve. Cancer Biology & Medicine. 2016;**13**(2):171-193

[3] Moreira RS, Bicker J, Musicco F, et al. Anti-PD-1 immunotherapy in advanced metastatic melanoma: State of the art and future challenges. Life Science. 2020;**240**:117433

[4] Kirkwood JM, Strawderman MH, Ernstoff MS, et al. Interferon alfa-2b adjuvant therapy of high-risk resected cutaneous melanoma: The Eastern Cooperative Oncology Group Trial EST 1684. Journal of Clinical Oncology. 1996;**14**:7-17

[5] Creagan ET, Ahmann DL, Frytak S, et al. Recombinant leukocyte A interferon (rIFN-aA) in the treatment of disseminated malignant melanoma. Analysis of complete and long-term responding patients. Cancer. 1986;**58**:2576-2578

[6] Tarhini AA, Gogas H, Kirkwood JM. IFN-α in the treatment of melanoma. Journal of Immunology. 2012;**189**(8):3789-3793

[7] Suciu S, Eggermont AMM, Lorigan P, et al. Relapse-free survival as a surrogate for overall survival in the evaluation of stage II-III Melanoma Adjuvant Therapy. Journal of the National Cancer Institute. 2018;**110**:1

[8] Rosenberg SA. IL-2: The first effective immunotherapy for human cancer. Journal of Immunology. 2014;**192**(12):5451-5458

[9] Atkins MB, Lotze MT, Dutcher JP, et al. High-dose recombinant interleukin 2 therapy for patients with metastatic melanoma: Analysis of 270 patients treated between 1985 and 1993. Journal of Clinical Oncology. 1999;**17**(7):2105-2116

[10] Kim DW, Gershenwald JE, Patel SP, Davies MA, Melanoma. In: The MD Anderson Manual of Medical Oncology. 3rd edition. McGraw-Hill Education; 2016. pp. 857-873

[11] Rosenberg SA, Lotze MT, Muul LM, et al. Observations on the systemic administration of autologous lymphokine-activated killer cells and recombinant interleukin-2 to patients with metastatic cancer. The New England Journal of Medicine. 1985;**313**:1485-1492

[12] Garbe C, Eigentler TK, Keilholz U, et al. Systematic review of medical treatment in melanoma: Current status and future prospects. The Oncologist. 2011;**16**(1):5-24

[13] Strub T, Ballotti R, Bertolotto C. The "ART" of epigenetics in melanoma: From histone "Alterations, to Resistance and Therapies". Theranostics. 2020;**10**(4):1777-1797

[14] Gross JA, Callas E, Allison JP. Identification and distribution of the costimulatory receptor CD28 in the mouse. Journal of Immunology. 1992;**149**(2):380-388

[15] Leach DR, Krummel MF, Allison JP. Enhancement of antitumor immunity by CTLA-4 blockade. Science. 1996;**271**(5256):1734-1736

[16] Ishida Y, Agata Y, Shibahara K, Honjo T. Induced expression of PD-1, a

novel member of the immunoglobulin gene superfamily, upon programmed cell death. The EMBO Journal. 1992;**11**:3887-3895

[17] Agata Y, Kawasaki A, Nishimura H, et al. Expression of the PD-1 antigen on the surface of stimulated mouse T and B lymphocytes. International Immunology. 1996;**8**(5):765-772

[18] Hodi FS, O'Day SJ, McDermott DF, et al. Improved survival with ipilimumab in patients with metastatic melanoma. The New England Journal of Medicine. 2010;**363**(8):711-723

[19] Robert C, Thomas L, Bondarenko I, et al. Ipilimumab plus dacarbazine for previously untreated metastatic melanoma. The New England Journal of Medicine. 2011;**364**(26):2517-2526

[20] Ascierto PA, Del Vecchio M, Robert C, et al. Ipilimumab 10 mg/kg versus ipilimumab 3 mg/kg in patients with unresectable or metastatic melanoma: A randomised, double-blind, multicentre, phase 3 trial. The Lancet Oncology. 2017;**18**(5):611-622

[21] Schadendorf D, Hodi FS, Robert C, et al. Pooled analysis of long-term survival data from Phase II and Phase III Trials of Ipilimumab in Unresectable or Metastatic Melanoma. Journal of Clinical Oncology. 2015;**33**(17):1889-1894

[22] Maio M, Grob JJ, Aamdal S, et al. Five-year survival rates for treatment-naive patients with advanced melanoma who received ipilimumab plus dacarbazine in a phase III trial. Journal of Clinical Oncology. 2015;**33**(10):1191-1196

[23] Krajsová I, Arenberger P, Lakomý R, et al. Long-term survival with Ipilimumab: Experience from a National Expanded Access Program for Patients with Melanoma. Anticancer Research. 2015;**35**(11):6303-6310

[24] Ascierto PA, Simeone E, Sileni VC, et al. Clinical experience with ipilimumab 3 mg/kg: Real-world efficacy and safety data from an expanded access programme cohort. Journal of Translational Medicine. 2014;**7**(12):116

[25] Wilgenhof S, Du Four S, Vandenbroucke F, et al. Single-center experience with ipilimumab in an expanded access program for patients with pretreated advanced melanoma. Journal of Immunotherapy. 2013;**36**(3):215-222

[26] Wiater K, Switaj T, Mackiewicz J, et al. Efficacy and safety of ipilimumab therapy in patients with metastatic melanoma: A retrospective multicenter analysis. Contemp Oncol (Pozn). 2013;**17**(3):257-262

[27] Jinga DC, Ciuleanu T, Negru S, et al. Effectiveness and safety profile of ipilimumab therapy in previously treated patients with unresectable or metastatic melanoma - the Romanian Patient Access Program. Journal of BUON. 2017;**22**(5):1287-1295

[28] Berrocal A, Arance A, Lopez Martin JA, et al. Ipilimumab for advanced melanoma: Experience from the Spanish Expanded Access Program. Melanoma Research. 2014;**24**(6):577-583

[29] Rapoport BL, Vorobiof DA, Dreosti LM, et al. Ipilimumab in pretreated patients with advanced malignant melanoma: Results of the South African Expanded-Access Program. Journal of Global Oncology. 2016;**3**(5):515-523

[30] Ahmad SS, Qian W, Ellis S, et al. Ipilimumab in the real world: The UK expanded access programme experience

in previously treated advanced melanoma patients. Melanoma Research. 2015;**25**(5):432-442

[31] Yervoy (Ipilimumab) prescribing information; revised May 2020: https://www.accessdata.fda.gov/drugsatfda_docs/label/2020/125377s110lbl.pdf

[32] Ribas A, Camacho LH, Lopez-Berestein G, et al. Antitumor activity in melanoma and anti-self responses in a phase I trial with the anti-cytotoxic T lymphocyte-associated antigen 4 monoclonal antibody CP-675,206. Journal of Clinical Oncology. 2005;**23**(35):8968-8977

[33] Ribas A, Kefford R, Marshall MA, et al. Phase III randomized clinical trial comparing tremelimumab with standard-of-care chemotherapy in patients with advanced melanoma. Journal of Clinical Oncology. 2013;**31**(5):616-622

[34] Daud A, Nandoskar P. Pembrolizumab for melanoma-safety profile and future trends. Expert Opinion on Drug Safety. 2016;**15**(6):727-729

[35] Robert C, Ribas A, Wolchok JD, et al. Anti-programmed-death-receptor-1 treatment with pembrolizumab in ipilimumab-refractory advanced melanoma: A randomised dose-comparison cohort of a phase 1 trial. Lancet. 2014;**384**(9948):1109-1117

[36] Ribas A, Puzanov I, Dummer R, et al. Pembrolizumab versus investigator-choice chemotherapy for ipilimumab-refractory melanoma (KEYNOTE-002): A randomised, controlled, phase 2 trial. The Lancet Oncology. 2015;**16**(8):908-918

[37] Hamid O, Puzanov I, Dummer R, et al. Final analysis of a randomised trial comparing pembrolizumab versus investigator-choice chemotherapy for ipilimumab-refractory advanced melanoma. European Journal of Cancer. 2017;**86**:37-45

[38] Schadendorf D, Dummer R, Hauschild A, et al. Health-related quality of life in the randomised KEYNOTE-002 study of pembrolizumab versus chemotherapy in patients with ipilimumab-refractory melanoma. European Journal of Cancer. 2016;**67**:46-54

[39] NCCN. Melanoma: Cutaneous; version 3.2022; April 11, 2022; https://www.nccn.org/

[40] Michielin O, Akkoi ACJ, Ascierto PA, et al. Cutaneous melanoma: ESMO Clinical Practice Guidelines for diagnosis, treatment and follow-up. Annals of Oncology. 2019;**30**:1184-1901

[41] Robert C, Schachter J, Long GV. et al; KEYNOTE-006 investigators. Pembrolizumab versus Ipilimumab in Advanced Melanoma. The New England Journal of Medicine. 2015;**372**(26):2521-2532

[42] Schachter J, Ribas A, Long GV, et al. Pembrolizumab versus ipilimumab for advanced melanoma: Final overall survival results of a multicentre, randomised, open-label phase 3 study (KEYNOTE-006). Lancet. 2017;**390**(10105):1853-1862

[43] Robert C, Ribas A, Hamid O, et al. Durable complete response after discontinuation of pembrolizumab in patients with metastatic melanoma. Journal of Clinical Oncology. 2018;**36**(17):1668-1674

[44] Weber JS, D'Angelo SP, Minor D, et al. Nivolumab versus chemotherapy in patients with advanced melanoma who progressed after anti-CTLA-4 treatment (CheckMate 037): A randomised, controlled, open-label, phase 3 trial. The Lancet Oncology. 2015;**16**(4):375-384

[45] Larkin J, Minor D, D'Angelo S, et al. Overall survival in patients with advanced melanoma who received nivolumab versus Investigator's Choice Chemotherapy in CheckMate 037: A Randomized, Controlled, Open-Label Phase III Trial. Journal of Clinical Oncology. 2018;**36**(4):383-390

[46] Robert C, Long GV, Brady B, et al. Nivolumab in previously untreated melanoma without BRAF mutation. The New England Journal of Medicine. 2015;**372**(4):320-330

[47] Ascierto PA, Long GV, Robert C, et al. Survival outcomes in patients with previously untreated BRAF wild-type advanced melanoma treated with nivolumab therapy: Three-Year Follow-up of a Randomized Phase 3 Trial. JAMA Oncology. 2019;**5**(2):187-194

[48] Hodi FS, Chiarion-Sileni V, Gonzalez R, et al. Nivolumab plus ipilimumab or nivolumab alone versus ipilimumab alone in advanced melanoma (CheckMate 067): 4-year outcomes of a multicentre, randomised, phase 3 trial. The Lancet Oncology. 2018;**19**(11):1480-1492

[49] Larkin J, Chiarion-Sileni V, Gonzalez R, et al. Combined Nivolumab and Ipilimumab or Monotherapy in Untreated Melanoma. The New England Journal of Medicine. 2015;**373**(1):23-34

[50] Wolchok JD, Chiarion-Sileni V, Gonzalez R, et al. overall survival with combined nivolumab and ipilimumab in advanced melanoma. The New England Journal of Medicine. 2017;**377**(14):1345-1356

[51] Curran MA, Montalvo W, Yagita H, Allison JP. PD-1 and CTLA-4 combination blockade expands infiltrating T cells and reduces regulatory T and myeloid cells within B16 melanoma tumors. Proceedings of the National Academy of Sciences of the United States of America. 2010;**107**(9):4275-4280

[52] Wolchok JD, Kluger H, Callahan MK, et al. Nivolumab plus ipilimumab in advanced melanoma. New England Journal of Medicine. 2013;**369**(2):122-133

[53] Hodi FS, Chesney J, Pavlick AC, et al. Combined nivolumab and ipilimumab versus ipilimumab alone in patients with advanced melanoma: 2-year overall survival outcomes in a multicentre, randomised, controlled, phase 2 trial. The Lancet Oncology. 2016;**17**(11):1558-1568

[54] Wolchok JD, Chiarion-Sileni V, Gonzalez R, et al. Long-term outcomes with nivolumab plus ipilimumab or nivolumab alone versus ipilimumab in patients with advanced melanoma. Journal of Clinical Oncology. 2022;**40**(2):127-137

[55] Schadendorf D, Wolchok JD, Hodi FS, et al. Efficacy and safety outcomes in patients with advanced melanoma who discontinued treatment with nivolumab and ipilimumab because of adverse events: A Pooled Analysis of Randomized Phase II and III Trials. Journal of Clinical Oncology. 2017;**35**(34):3807-3814

[56] Daud AI, Wolchok JD, Robert C, et al. Programmed death-ligand 1 expression and response to the anti-programmed Death 1 Antibody Pembrolizumab in Melanoma. Journal of Clinical Oncology. 2016;**34**(34):4102-4109

[57] Andtbacka RH, Kaufman HL, Collichio F, et al. Talimogene laherparepvec improves durable response rate in patients with advanced melanoma. Journal of Clinical Oncology. 2015;**33**(25):2780-2788

[58] Chesney J, Puzanov I, Collichio F, et al. Randomized, Open-Label Phase II Study Evaluating the Efficacy and Safety of Talimogene Laherparepvec in Combination With Ipilimumab Versus Ipilimumab Alone in Patients With Advanced, Unresectable Melanoma. Journal of Clinical Oncology. 2018;**36**(17):1658-1667

[59] Long G, Dummer R, Andtbacka R, et al. Follow-up analysis of MASTERKEY-265 Phase 1b (ph1b) trial of talimogene laherparepvec (T-VEC) in combination (combo) with pembrolizumab (pembro) in patients (pts) with unresectable stage IIIB–IVM1c melanoma (MEL). Pigment Cell & Melanoma Research. 2019;**32**:133-134

[60] Margolin K, Ernstoff MS, Hamid O, et al. Ipilimumab in patients with melanoma and brain metastases: An open-label, phase 2 trial. The Lancet Oncology. 2012;**13**(5):459-465

[61] Kluger HM, Chiang V, Mahajan A, et al. Long-term survival of patients with melanoma with active brain metastases treated with pembrolizumab on a Phase II Trial. Journal of Clinical Oncology. 2019;**37**(1):52-60

[62] Long GV, Atkinson V, Lo S, et al. Combination nivolumab and ipilimumab or nivolumab alone in melanoma brain metastases: A multicentre randomised phase 2 study. The Lancet Oncology. 2018;**19**(5):672-681

[63] Tawbi HA, Forsyth PA, Algazi A, et al. Combined Nivolumab and Ipilimumab in Melanoma Metastatic to the Brain. The New England Journal of Medicine. 2018;**379**(8):722-730

[64] Minniti G, Anzellini D, Reverberi C, et al. Stereotactic radiosurgery combined with nivolumab or Ipilimumab for patients with melanoma brain metastases: Evaluation of brain control and toxicity. Journal for Immunotherapy of Cancer. 2019;**7**(1):102

[65] Zimmer L, Apuri S, Eroglu Z, et al. Ipilimumab alone or in combination with nivolumab after progression on anti-PD-1 therapy in advanced melanoma. European Journal of Cancer. 2017;**75**:47-55

[66] Pires da Silva I, Ahmed T, Reijers ILM, et al. Ipilimumab alone or ipilimumab plus anti-PD-1 therapy in patients with metastatic melanoma resistant to anti-PD-(L)1 monotherapy: A multicentre, retrospective, cohort study. The Lancet Oncology. 2021;**22**(6):836-847

[67] Taylor MH, Lee CH, Makker V, et al. Phase IB/II Trial of Lenvatinib plus pembrolizumab in patients with advanced renal cell carcinoma, endometrial cancer, and other selected advanced solid tumors. Journal of Clinical Oncology. 2020;**38**(11):1154-1163

[68] Miranda C, Mazzoni M, Sensi M, Pierotti MA, Greco A. Functional characterization of NTRK1 mutations identified in melanoma. Genes, Chromosomes & Cancer. 2020;**53**:875-880

[69] Curti BD, Faries MB. Recent advances in the treatment of melanoma. The New England Journal of Medicine. 2021;**384**(23):2229-2240

[70] Ugurel S, Röhmel J, Ascierto PA, et al. Survival of patients with advanced metastatic melanoma: The impact of novel therapies. European Journal of Cancer. 2016;**53**:125-134

[71] Pasquali S, Hadjinicolaou AV, Chiarion Sileni V, et al. Systemic treatments for metastatic cutaneous

melanoma. Cochrane Database of Systematic Reviews. 2018;**2**:CD011123

[72] Dummer R, Ascierto PA, Gogas HJ, et al. Encorafenib plus binimetinib versus vemurafenib or encorafenib in patients with BRAF-mutant melanoma (COLUMBUS): A multicentre, open-label, randomised phase 3 trial. The Lancet Oncology. 2018;**19**(5):603-615

[73] Jansen YJL, Rozeman EA, Mason R, et al. Discontinuation of anti-PD-1 antibody therapy in the absence of disease progression or treatment limiting toxicity: Clinical outcomes in advanced melanoma. Annals of Oncology. 2019;**30**(7):1154-1161

[74] Ascierto PA, Mandala M, Ferrucci PF, et al. SECOMBIT: The best sequential approach with combo immunotherapy [ipilimumab (I) /nivolumab (N)] and combo target therapy [encorafenib (E)/ binimetinib (B)] in patients with BRAF mutated metastatic melanoma: A phase II randomized study; abstract LBA40, presented at ESMO Congress. 2021

[75] Atkins MB, Lee SJ, Chmielowski B, et al. DREAMseq (Doublet, Randomized Evaluation in Advanced Melanoma Sequencing): A phase III trial—ECOG-ACRIN EA6134. Journal of Clinical Oncology. 2021;**39**:36

[76] Keilholz U, Ascierto PA, Dummer R, et al. ESMO consensus conference recommendations on the management of metastatic melanoma: Under the auspices of the ESMO Guidelines Committe. Annals of Oncology. 2020;**31**(11):1435-1448

[77] Hamid O, Robert C, Daud A, et al. Five-year survival outcomes for patients with advanced melanoma treated with pembrolizumab in KEYNOTE-001. Annals of Oncology. 2019;**30**(4): 582-588

[78] Hepner A, Versluis JM, Gerard CL, et al. The nature and management of acquired resistance to PD1-based therapy in melanoma. Journal of Clinical Oncology. 2020;**38**:10014-10014

[79] Moreira A, Heinzerling L. Current melanoma treatments: Where do we stand? Cancers. 2021;**13**:221

[80] Bhave P, Pallan L, Long GV, et al. Melanoma recurrence patterns and management after adjuvant targeted therapy: A multicentre analysis. British Journal of Cancer. 2021;**124**:574-580

[81] Wang DY, Salem JE, Cohen JV, et al. Fatal toxic effects associated with immune checkpoint inhibitors: A systematic review and meta-analysis. JAMA. 2021;**4124**:1721-1728

[82] NCCN. Management of Immunotherapy-related toxicities version 1.2022-February 28, 2022; https://www.nccn.org/

[83] Weber JS, Hodi FS, Wolchok JD, et al. Safety profile of nivolumab monotherapy: A pooled analysis of patients with advanced melanoma. Journal of Clinical Oncology. 2017;**35**(7):785-792

[84] Sznol M, Ferrucci PF, Hogg D, et al. Pooled analysis safety profile of nivolumab and ipilimumab combination therapy in patients with advanced melanoma. Journal of Clinical Oncology. 2017;**35**(34):3815-3822

[85] Iida N, Dzutsev A, Stewart CA, et al. Commensal bacteria control cancer response to therapy by modulating the tumor microenvironment. Science. 2013;**342**(6161):967-970

[86] Pinato DJ, Howlett S, Ottaviani D, et al. Association of prior antibiotic treatment with survival and response to

immune checkpoint inhibitor therapy in patients with cancer. JAMA Oncology. 2019;**5**(12):1774-1778

[87] Lythgoe MP, Liu DSK, Annels NE, et al. Gene of the month: Lymphocyte-activation gene 3 (LAG-3). Jpurnal of Clinical Patholhplogy. 2021;**74**:543-547

[88] Tawbi HA, Schadendorf D, Lipson EJ, et al. Relatlimab andnivolumab versus nivolumab in untreated advanced melanoma. New England Journal of Medicine. 2022;**386**:24-34

[89] Frampton AE, Sivakumar S. A new combination immunotherapy in advanced melanoma. New England Journal of Medicine. 2022;**386**:91-92

[90] Powderly J, Patel MR, Lee JJ, et al. CA-170, a first in class oral small molecule dual inhibitor of immune checkpoints PD-L1 and VISTA, demonstrates tumor growth inhibition in pre-clinical models and promotes T cell activation in Phase 1 study. Cancer. 2017;**28**:V405-V406

[91] Acharya N, Sabatos-Peyton C, Anderson AC. Tim-3 finds its place in the cancer immunotherapy landscape. Journal for Immunotherapy of Cancer. 2020;**8**(1):e000911

[92] Diab A, Tykodi SS, Daniels GA, et al. Bempegaldesleukin plus nivolumab in first-line metastatic melanoma. Journal of Clinical Oncology. 2021;**39**(26):2914-2925

[93] Switzer B, Puzanov I, Skitzki JJ, et al. Managing metastatic melanoma in 2022: A clinical review. Journal of Clinical Oncology. 2022;**18**(5):335-351

[94] Goff SL, Dudley ME, Citrin DE, et al. Randomized, prospective evaluation comparing intensity of lymphodepletion before adoptive transfer of tumor-infiltrating lymphocytes for patients with metastatic melanoma. Journal of Clinical Oncology. 2016;**34**(20):2389-2397

[95] Sarnaik AA, Hamid O, Khushalani NI, et al. Lifileucel, a tumor-infiltrating lymphocyte therapy, in metastatic melanoma. Journal of Clinical Oncology. 2021;**39**(24):2656-2666

Section 6

Challenges in Melanoma: Intracraneal Metastases and Uveal Melanoma

Chapter 7

Uveal Melanoma: Factors Determining Metastatic Process, Epidemiology, Diagnosis, and Treatment

Darina Lysková, Paulína Plesníková,
Viera Horvathova Kajabova, Lucia Demkova,
Božena Smolková and Jela Valášková

Abstract

Uveal melanoma (UM) is an ocular tumor with a dismal prognosis. It is the most frequent primary intraocular tumor in adults. The primary goal of treatment for uveal melanomas is to prevent metastasis. Despite outstanding advances in the diagnosis and treatment of primary UM, nearly 50% of patients develop metastases via hematogenous dissemination. Estimation of prognosis for patients with UM can be achieved by detecting genetic alterations or epigenetic changes in the tumor tissues. However, these techniques are not always available. The clinicopathological characteristics with limited accuracy are widely used instead to predict metastatic potential. Identifying novel markers with prognostic potential can help refine the prognosis of UM patients. As we know, no existing therapy has a significantly better impact on preventing metastasis. Based on published theories, the key role is existing micrometastasis before therapy starts. Researchers are focusing on developing adjuvant systemic therapy for metastatic UM. Getting to know the cause of metastatic uveal melanoma is crucial in it.

Keywords: uveal melanoma, metastases, genetic changes in UM, epigenetic changes in UM, epidemiology of UM, diagnosis and treatment UM

1. Introduction

Uveal melanoma is a rare form of melanoma, but the most frequent intraocular tumor in adults [1]. Comprising approximately 83% of ocular and 3% of all melanomas. It arises from melanocytes along the uveal layer of the eye, including the iris, ciliary body, and most often the choroid [2].

Primary UM is treated with either surgery or radiation with a low local recurrence rate. However, almost half of UM patients develop metastases, which may be caused by a virtually undetectable neoplasm already present at the time of the primary tumor diagnosis [3]. Most UM patients survive less than 12 months after metastases diagnosis due to the lack of effective therapies [4]. UM spreads through the blood. The liver is the preferred metastatic site, followed by the lungs and bones [5].

Various clinical, pathological, molecular, and cytogenetic markers assessed in tumors, such as specific chromosome copy number alterations [6], gene expression profiles [7], and the mutation status of known UM driver genes [8], can predict the risk of metastases and survival.

2. Genetic changes in uveal melanoma

2.1 Chromosomal rearrangements

The most frequent UM-specific aberrations include monosomy of chromosome 3 (M3), a gain in the short arm of chromosome 6 (6p), or a gain in the long arm of chromosome 8 (8q). Similar to the loss of the short arm of chromosome 8 (8p), the long arm of chromosome 6 (6q), and the short arm of chromosome 1 (1p) pose a high metastatic risk and present a poor prognosis [9–11].

Conversely, the presence of 6p amplification represents a protective factor due to its association with a good prognosis and lowered metastatic risk [12]. Although their prognostic value has been proven, and their sensitivity and specificity are limited in clinical use [13]. The problem seems to be that results differ based on laboratory methods used for detecting the amount of chromosomal copies, and they are not accurate.

2.2 Change in gene expression

Another way to predict the risk of metastasis is via gene expression analysis. A commercially available expression panel of 15 genes developed by Castle Biosciences categorizes patients as Class 1 (low metastatic risk) or Class 2 transcriptional subtype (high metastatic risk) [7, 14]. Four molecular subsets were proposed recently, based on a more complex classification [15, 16].

2.3 Mutation of genes

UM occurs mostly sporadically, however, rarely it occurs in families with an inherited predisposition for this malignancy. Mutations in gene BAP 1 are segregated in an autosomal dominant manner in the hereditary tumor syndrome. It is characterized by the occurrence of tumor disease in a family member at a young age, by the presence of numerous primary tumors, often bilaterally when the steam organs are affected. BAP 1 mutation is associated with cutaneous melanoma, mesothelioma, meningioma, and many others. The clinical phenotype includes UM in patients with oculodermal melanocytosis, skin melanoma, neurofibromatosis type 1, and Li-Fraumeni syndrome. In the case of a familiar form, the combination of clinical signs and genetic information can be used for early diagnosis in patients [17–19].

3. Epigenetics in uveal melanoma

The term epigenetics includes changes in gene expression and chromatin structure that are not related to a change in primary genetic information, that is, changes not encoded in the sequence of bases in the DNA chain [20]. In the broadest sense of the word, epigenetics can be understood as a bridge between the genotype and the phenotype of a cell [21].

The basic epigenetic mechanisms of gene expression regulation include DNA methylation, histone modification with subsequent chromatin remodeling, and non-coding RNA [22]. These mechanisms are essential for the normal development and homeostasis of the organism, and their disruption can lead to changes in gene function and malignant transformation, and can have an impact on individual signaling pathways involved in metastasis [23].

Epigenetic inactivation plays a role in genes located on chromosomes 1, 3, 6, or 8, that is, in chromosomes with proven abnormalities in UM. Monosomy 3 is present in approximately half of patients with UM. Genes that play a key role in hematogenous dissemination are located on this chromosome, for example, BAP1, RASSF1A, FHIT, CTNNB1, and SRY.

3.1 Methylation

It is the binding of a methyl group (-CH3) to the fifth carbon of cytosine by a covalent bond. Compared to normal cells, tumor cells have a disturbed DNA methylation pattern either by decreasing (hypomethylation) or increasing (hypermethylation) the number of methyl groups. During the onset of oncological diseases, these are significant processes that lead to an increase in chromosome instability. Primarily hypermethylation of promoters of tumor suppressor genes, hypomethylation of proto-oncogenes, and global hypomethylation [24].

In UM patients, DNA methylation was identified as the cause of inactivation of several genes. Aberrant hypomethylation of the PRAME gene, leading to its transcriptional inactivation, was associated with an increased metastatic risk [25]. The majority of hypermethylated genes in UM are p16, TIMP3, RASSF1A, RASEF, hTERT, and ES genes. They participate in the regulation of the cell cycle. Only the RASSF1A and p16 genes are also methylated in skin melanoma. In comparison, genes methylated in cutaneous melanoma, such as pTEN, TNFSF10D, COL1A2, MAGE, or CLDN11, were not methylated in UM [26].

Decreased levels of E-cadherin, a key protein that is inhibited in the epithelial-mesenchymal transition process, were identified in 56.2% of UM. They were indirectly correlated with the methylation of the CDH1 promoter gene, which encodes it [27, 28].

The researchers induced an increase in the expression of E-cadherin, which affected the phenotypic change in UM cells from spindle cell to epithelial type. Reactivation of the expression of aberrantly methylated genes by DNMTs inhibitors may represent a promising therapeutic strategy [23].

3.2 modifikácie histónov

Histones are basic proteins abundant in lysine and arginine residues that are found in nuclei of eukaryotic cells. They create structural units called nucleosomes. We know five families of histones H1/H5 (linker histones), H2, H3, and H4 (core histones). The nucleosome core is formed of two H2A–H2B dimers and a H3–H4 tetramer. Nucleosomes are wrapped into fibers of tightly packed chromatin. That means DNA winds around them. Histones prevent DNA from becoming tangled and protect it from DNA damage. They play important roles in DNA replication and gene regulation [29].

Post-translational covalent changes occur at the N-terminal ends of histones in mammalian cells through the action of histone-modifying enzymes. The most common modifications of histones, which play a key role in the regulation of gene expression are methylation, acetylation, phosphorylation, and ubiquitination. They affect the mobility and stability of chromatin and regulate its transcription [23].

Most UM Class 2 transcriptional subtype (high metastatic risk) contains inactivating mutations of the tumor suppressor gene BAP1. It encodes bap 1, which has a role in the progression of UM. It modifies histones by catalyzing the removal of ubiquitin from histone H2A. Its depletion leads to hyperubiquitination of H2A in melanocytes and melanoma cells and subsequent loss of differentiation and acquisition of tumor stem cell properties [30].

Histone deacetylase inhibitors (HDAC), therefore enable the restoration of the expression of epigenetically inactivated genes, necessary, for example, to control the cell cycle. In UM cell lines, primocultures created from patient tumor cells, and HDAC inhibitors, such as valproic acid, trichostatin A, panobinostat LBH-589, and suberoylanilide hydroxamic acid-induced proliferation inhibition, cell cycle arrest, increased tumor cell apoptosis, morphological and transcriptional changes consistent with melanocyte differentiation. HDAC inhibitors are in preclinical studies for the treatment of UM with the aim of prolonging the dormancy of micrometastatic disease [31, 32].

3.3 Non-coding mRNA

MicroRNA (miRNA) is mainly considered non-coding mRNA. These are short nucleotide single-stranded RNA molecules that participate in the post-transcriptional regulation of the expression of mediator RNAs (mRNA). It has been proven that miRNA functions as an oncogene or tumor suppressor gene in carcinogenesis. It binds to complementary mRNA and thereby inhibits mRNA translation and inactivates target genes [33].

Changes in the expression of many miRNAs have been described in cell lines of tumor structures and peripheral blood from patients with UM [34]. They play an important role in the deregulation of oncogenic pathways in UM and may promote metastatic spread. In addition to the fact that miRNAs can be interesting diagnostic and prognostic biomarkers, they offer us new therapeutic targets [35].

Epigenetic changes play an important role in the pathogenesis of oncological diseases. They are reversible; therefore, they are a good therapeutic target. In many preclinical studies, it has been proven that epigenetic drugs enable the restoration of aberrantly inactivated tumor-suppressor genes, and increase the sensitivity of resistant tumor cells to treatment.

The prerequisite for the discovery of effective drugs for the adjuvant therapy of UM and the treatment of metastatic UM is to necessarily accept the importance of epigenetic changes and understand their role in the pathogenesis of this disease.

4. Epidemiology

The most common primary intraocular malignancy in adults is uveal melanoma. It arises from melanocytes in the choroid, ciliary body, or iris. The incidence is 5.1 per million and has remained stable since at least 1970s. UM is the most common in Caucasians during the fifth to sixth decade of life [1]. Approximately 85% of UM is localized in the choroid [36], about 4–7% in the ciliary body, and 2–4% in iris, which is associated with early diagnosis and the best prognosis [37]. Associated with the worst prognosis is UM in the ciliary body.

5. Clinical diagnosis

Physical examination and health history are used to help diagnose intraocular melanoma, as well as eye exam with the dilated pupil (by ophthalmoscopy or slit-lamp biomicroscopy). Diagnosing uveal melanoma often requires serial fundus photography. Fluorescein angiography or indocyanine green angiography is used in the screening and follow-up of suspicious lesions. Other critical tools in the diagnosis of uveal melanoma are A and B scan ultrasonography and optical coherence tomography.

6. Management

The primary goal of treatment for uveal melanomas is to prevent metastasis. However, treatment of small lesions (less than 3 mm in thickness) is controversial, and it is not proven whether it prevents metastasis. Observation is generally recommended whenever it is possible.

Biopsy of the lesion is the only way to definitively identify uveal melanoma. It can be done after enucleation or by fine needle aspiration biopsy. The collected material is used for histological examination and cytopathological analysis.

Historically, enucleation (eyeball removal) was the standard treatment for primary UM, and it is still used when large tumors are present. However, it has been largely replaced by radiation therapy (i.e., brachytherapy or proton beam therapy) to spare the affected eye.

The results of the Collaborative Ocular Melanoma Study (COMS) in 2001, a large multicenter randomized control trial with 1317 patients confirmed that there was no significant difference in mortality after brachytherapy in comparison to enucleation for malignant UM [38]. Later other publications reported similar positive findings [39–41]. The decision to use brachytherapy vs. proton beam therapy is now largely made in regard to the size and location of the tumor and patient preference [42–45]. Secondary complication can be present as glaucoma, serous retinal detachment, or cataract. The only effective treatment for cataracts is surgery with precise intra ocular lens power calculation [46, 47]. The serous retinal detachment can be present as complication in whole scale of eye disease, for example, uveal effusion syndrome [48].

For small tumors, the less commonly available treatment options can be used. These include transpupillary thermotherapy, photocoagulation, photodynamic therapy, and local resection.

Acknowledgement

Our publication was supported by APVV-17-0369 and VEGA 1/0395/21 projects.

Conflict of interest

The authors declare no conflict of interest.

Appendices and nomenclature

UM	Uveal melanoma
BAP 1	BRCA1 associated protein 1
RASSF1	Ras association domain family member 1
FHIT 2	Fragile Histidine Triad Diadenosine Triphosphatase 2
CTNNB 1	Catenin Cadherin-Associated Protein Beta 1
SRY, SOX2	Sex determining region Y-box 2
PRAME	Nuclear Receptor Transcriptional Regulator
p16, CDKN2A	Cyclin-dependent kinase inhibitor 2A
TIMP3	TIMP metallopeptidase inhibitor 3
RASSF1	Ras association domain family member 1
RASEF	RAS And EF-Hand Domain Containing
hTERT	Telomerase reverse transcriptase in humans
PTEN	Phosphatase and tensin homolog
TNFSF10D	Tumor necrosis factor receptor super family member 10D
COL1A2	Collagen Type I Alpha 2 Chain
MAGE	The Melanoma Antigen Gene
CLDN11	Claudin 11
DNMTs	DNA methyltransferases
CDH1	Cadherin 1
HDAC	Histone deacetylase inhibitors

Author details

Darina Lysková[1,2]*, Paulína Plesníková[1,2], Viera Horvathova Kajabova[3], Lucia Demkova[3], Božena Smolková[3] and Jela Valášková[1]

1 Faculty of Medicine, Department of Ophthalmology, Comenius University in Bratislava, Slovakia

2 Faculty of Medicine, Comenius University, Bratislava, Slovakia

3 Cancer Research Institute, Biomedical Research Center, Slovak Academy of Sciences, Bratislava, Slovakia

*Address all correspondence to: darina.lyskova@gmail.com

References

[1] Singh AD, Turell ME, Topham AK. Uveal melanoma: Trends in incidence, treatment, and survival. Ophthalmology. 2011;**118**(9):1881-1885. DOI: 10.1016/j.ophtha.2011.01.040

[2] McLaughlin CC, Wu XC, Jemal A, Martin HJ, Roche LM, Chen VW. Incidence of noncutaneous melanomas in the U.S. Cancer. 2005;**103**(5):1000-1007. DOI: 10.1002/cncr.20866

[3] Eskelin S, Pyrhönen S, Summanen P, Hahka-Kemppinen M, Kivelä T. Tumor doubling times in metastatic malignant melanoma of the uvea: Tumor progression before and after treatment. Ophthalmology. 2000;**107**:1443-1449. DOI: 10.1016/S0161-6420(00)00182-2

[4] Blum ES, Yang J, Komatsubara KM, Carvajal RD. Clinical management of uveal and conjunctival melanoma. Oncology (Williston Park). 2016;**30**(1):29-48

[5] Diener-West M, Reynolds SM, Agugliaro DJ, et al. Development of metastatic disease after enrollment in the COMS trials for treatment of choroidal melanoma: Collaborative Ocular Melanoma Study Group Report No. 26. Archives of Ophthalmology. 2005;**123**(12):1639-1643. DOI: 10.1001/archopht.123.12.1639

[6] Damato B, Coupland SE. Translating uveal melanoma cytogenetics into clinical care. Archives of Ophthalmology. 2009;**127**(4):423-429. DOI: 10.1001/archophthalmol.2009.40

[7] Onken MD, Worley LA, Ehlers JP, Harbour JW. Gene expression profiling in uveal melanoma reveals two molecular classes and predicts metastatic death. Cancer Research. 2004;**64**(20):7205-7209. DOI: 10.1158/0008-5472.CAN-04-1750

[8] Johansson PA, Brooks K, Newell F, et al. Whole genome landscapes of uveal melanoma show an ultraviolet radiation signature in iris tumours. Nature Communications. 2020;**11**:2408. DOI: 10.1038/s41467-020-16276-8

[9] Ehlers JP, Worley L, Onken MD, Harbour JW. Integrative genomic analysis of aneuploidy in uveal melanoma. Clinical Cancer Research. 2008;**14**(1):115-122. DOI: 10.1158/1078-0432.CCR-07-1825

[10] Ewens KG, Kanetsky PA, Richards-Yutz J, et al. Genomic profile of 320 uveal melanoma cases: Chromosome 8p-loss and metastatic outcome. Investigative Ophthalmology & Visual Science. 2013;**54**(8):5721-5729. DOI: 10.1167/iovs.13-12195

[11] Versluis M, de Lange MJ, van Pelt SI, Ruivenkamp CAL, Kroes WGM, et al. Digital PCR validates 8q dosage as prognostic tool in uveal melanoma. PLoS One. 2015;**10**(3):e0116371. DOI: 10.1371/journal.pone.0116371

[12] Amaro A, Gangemi R, Piaggio F, et al. The biology of uveal melanoma. Cancer Metastasis Reviews. 2017;**36**: 109-140. DOI: 10.1007/s10555-017-9663-3

[13] Kaliki S, Shields CL, Shields J. Uveal melanoma. Indian Journal of Ophthalmology. 2015;**63**(2):93-102. DOI: 10.4103/0301-4738.154367

[14] Onken MD, Worley LA, Char DH, Augsburger JJ, Correa ZM, Nudleman E, et al. Collaborative ocular oncology group report number 1: Prospective validation of a multi-gene prognostic assay in

uveal melanoma. Ophthalmology. 2012;**119**:1596-1603. DOI: 10.1016/j.ophtha.2012.02.017

[15] Robertson AG, Shih J, Yau C, et al. Integrative analysis identifies four molecular and clinical subsets in uveal melanoma. Cancer Cell. 2017;**32**(2):204, e15-220. DOI: 10.1016/j.ccell.2017.07.003

[16] Jager MJ, Shields CL, Cebulla CM, et al. Uveal melanoma. Nature Reviews. Disease Primers. 2020;**6**(1):24. DOI: 10.1038/s41572-020-0158-0

[17] Houlston RS, Damato BE. Genetic predisposition to ocular melanoma. Eye (London, England). 1999;**13**(Pt 1):43-46. DOI: 10.1038/eye.1999.9

[18] Jay M, McCartney AC. Familial malignant melanoma of the uvea and p53: A Victorian detective story. Survey of Ophthalmology. 1993;**37**(6):457-462. DOI: 10.1016/0039-6257(93)90142-t

[19] Easton DF, Steele L, Fields P, et al. Cancer risks in two large breast cancer families linked to BRCA2 on chromosome 13q12-13. American Journal of Human Genetics. 1997;**61**(1):120-128. DOI: 10.1086/513891

[20] Herceg Z, Hainaut P. Genetic and epigenetic alterations as biomarkers for cancer detection, diagnosis and prognosis. Molecular Oncology. 2007;**1**(1):26-41. DOI: 10.1016/j.molonc.2007.01.004

[21] Bird A. DNA methylation patterns and epigenetic memory. Genes & Development. 2002;**16**(1):6-21. DOI: 10.1101/gad.947102

[22] Chokhachi Baradaran P, Kozovska Z, Furdova A, Smolkova B. Targeting epigenetic modifications in uveal melanoma. International Journal of Molecular Sciences. 2020;**21**(15):5314

[23] Sharma S, Kelly TK, Jones PA. Epigenetics in cancer. Carcinogenesis. 2010;**31**(1):27-36. DOI: 0.1093/carcin/bgp220

[24] Greenberg MVC, Bourc'his D. The diverse roles of DNA methylation in mammalian development and disease. Nature Reviews. Molecular Cell Biology. 2019;**20**(10):590-607. DOI: 10.1038/s41580-019-0159-6

[25] Field MG, Durante MA, Decatur CL, et al. Epigenetic reprogramming and aberrant expression of PRAME are associated with increased metastatic risk in class 1 and class 2 uveal melanomas. Oncotarget. 2016;**7**(37):59209-59219. DOI: 10.18632/oncotarget.10962

[26] Fu S, Wu H, Zhang H, Lian CG, Lu Q. DNA methylation/hydroxymethylation in melanoma. Oncotarget. 2017;**8**(44):78163-78173. DOI: 10.18632/oncotarget.18293

[27] Venza M, Visalli M, Catalano T, et al. DNA methylation-induced E-cadherin silencing is correlated with the clinicopathological features of melanoma. Oncology Reportsa. 2016;**35**(4):2451-2460. DOI: 10.3892/or.2016.4618

[28] Versluis M, De Lange MJ, Van Pelt S, Luzten GPM, Jager MJ. Epigenetic regulation of the epithelial phenotype in uveal melanoma. Acta Ophtalmology. 2013;**2**:5-8. DOI: 10.1111/j.1755-3768.2013.1773.x

[29] Kanwal R, Gupta S. Epigenetic modifications in cancer. Clinical Genetics. 2012;**81**(4):303-311. DOI: 10.1111/j.1399-0004.2011.01809.x

[30] Matatall KA, Agapova OA, Onken MD, Worley LA, Bowcock AM, Harbour JW. BAP1 deficiency causes loss of melanocytic cell identity in uveal

melanoma. BMC Cancer. 2013;**13**:371. DOI: 10.1186/1471-2407-13-371

[31] Landreville S, Agapova OA, Matatall KA, et al. Histone deacetylase inhibitors induce growth arrest and differentiation in uveal melanoma. Clinical Cancer Research. 2012;**18**(2):408-416. DOI: 10.1158/1078-0432.CCR-11-0946

[32] Moschos SJ, Mantzoros CS. The role of the IGF system in cancer: From basic to clinical studies and clinical applications. Oncology. 2002;**63**(4):317-332. DOI: 10.1159/000066230

[33] Piva R, Spandidos DA, Gambari R. From microRNA functions to microRNA therapeutics: Novel targets and novel drugs in breast cancer research and treatment (review). International Journal of Oncology. 2013;**43**(4):985-994. DOI: 10.3892/ijo.2013.2059

[34] Horvathova Kajabova V, Soltysova A, Demkova L, Plesnikova P, Lyskova D, Furdova A, et al. *KIT* expression is regulated by DNA methylation in uveal melanoma tumors. International Journal of Molecular Sciences. 2021;**22**(19):10748

[35] Smit KN, Chang J, Derks K, et al. Aberrant MicroRNA expression and its implications for uveal melanoma metastasis. Cancers (Basel). 2019;**11**(6):815. DOI: 10.3390/cancers11060815

[36] Shields CL, Kaliki S, Furuta M, Mashayekhi A, Shields JA. Clinical spectrum and prognosis of uveal melanoma based on age at presentation in 8,033 cases. Retina. 2012;**32**(7):1363-1372

[37] Shields CL, Kaliki S, Shah SU, Luo W, Furuta M, Shields JA. Iris melanoma: Features and prognosis in 317 children and adults. Journal of AAPOS. 2012;**16**(1):10-16

[38] Singh AD, Kalyani P, Topham A. Estimating the risk of malignant transformation of a choroidal nevus. Ophthalmology. 2005;**112**(10):1784-1789

[39] Furdova A, Sramka M, Chorvath M, Kralik G, Krasnik V, Krcova I, Waczulikova I. Stereotactic radiosurgery in intraocular malignant melanoma-retrospective study. Neuro Endocrinology Letters. Jan 2014;**35**(1):28-36

[40] Furdova A, Sramka M, Chorvath M, Kralik G, Furda R, Gregus M. Clinical experience of stereotactic radiosurgery at a linear accelerator for intraocular melanoma. Melanoma Research. Oct 2017;**27**(5):463-468

[41] Furdova A, Babal P, Kobzova D, Zahorjanova P, Kapitanova K, Sramka M, et al. Uveal melanoma survival rates after single dose stereotactic radiosurgery. Neoplasma. 15 Nov 2018;**65**(6):965-971

[42] Furdova A, Furda R, Sramka M, et al. Stereotactic irradiation on linear accelerator - ultrasound versus MRI in choroidal melanoma volume calculation. BMC Ophthalmology. 2022;**22**:333

[43] Zahorjanová P, Sekáč J, Babál P, Štubňa M. Enucleation after stereotactic radiosurgery in patients with uveal melanoma. Čes. a slov. Oftal. 2020;**76**(1):46-51

[44] Furdova A, Sramka M. Uveal Malignant Melanoma and Stereotactic Radiosurgery: Intraocular Uveal Melanoma and One-Day Session Stereotactic Radiosurgery at Linear Accelerator. Saarbrücken: LAP LAMBERT Academic Publishing; 2014. p. 188

[45] Horkovicova K, Furdova A. Uveal melanoma. In: Lasfar A,

Cohen-Solal K, editors. Melanoma. London, UK: IntechOpen; 2020

[46] Popov I, Waczulikova I, Stefanickova J, et al. Analysis of biometric parameters of 2340 eyes measured with optical biometer Lenstar LS900 in a Caucasian population. European Journal of Ophthalmology. 2022;**32**(1):213-220

[47] Popov I, Popova V, Sekac J, Krasnik V. Does every calculation formula fit for all types of intraocular lenses? Optimization of constants for Tecnis ZA9003 and ZCB00 is necessary. Medicina. 2021;**57**(4):319

[48] Popov I, Popova V, Krasnik V. Comparing the results of vitrectomy and sclerectomy in a patient with nanophthalmic uveal effusion syndrome. Medicina. 2021;**57**(2):120

Chapter 8

Intracranial Metastatic Melanoma

Hiu Kwan Carolyn Tang and Joon Wee Ho

Abstract

Central nervous system (CNS) metastases are a common manifestation of malignant melanoma, with a median overall survival of as little as 4.7 months based on a study of patients diagnosed between 1986 and 2004 prior to the era of effective systemic therapy. Yet most of the clinical trials exclude patients with intra-cranial metastases. CNS involvement often causes neurological deficits and functional impairment. Localised therapies, such as surgical excision and stereotactic radiotherapy are applicable to only a minority of patients. There are evidences of clinical benefits for immunotherapy than best supportive care and when given alongside radiotherapy provides a better overall survival than radiotherapy alone. This chapter evaluates the efficacy and toxicity of these treatments against advanced melanoma patients with brain metastases.

Keywords: melanoma, metastatic melanoma, melanoma brain metastases MBM, immunotherapy, radiotherapy, stereotactic radiotherapy, brain metastases, CNS metastases

1. Introduction

Central nervous system metastases are a common and often lethal manifestation of malignant melanoma, with a median overall survival of as little as 4.7 months based on a study of patients diagnosed between 1986 and 2004 prior to the era of effective systemic therapy [1]. Although both cutaneous and mucosal melanomas have a high propensity for CNS dissemination, this is almost unheard of with uveal melanoma despite the close anatomical proximity of the eye and brain [2]. CNS involvement often causes neurological deficits and functional impairment. Localised therapies, such as surgical excision and stereotactic radiotherapy, are applicable to only a minority of patients. However, stereotactic radiation therapy is able to overcome the relative radio-resistance of melanoma by delivering extremely high doses of radiotherapy with little damage to surrounding brain tissue [3]. It is also increasingly appreciated that stereotactic radiotherapy may drive immunogenic cell death and this can lead to regression of non-irradiated lesions via immune priming and the 'abscopal' effect [4]. Radiotherapy can upregulate tumoural PD-L1 expression and can lead to increased T-cell infiltration of tumours with increased proinflammatory cytokine levels [5, 6]. This potential synergistic interaction between stereotactic radiotherapy and immunotherapy could be exploited and this is being explored in current clinical trials (PERM trial NCT02562625). Symptomatic patients require corticosteroid therapy to reduce peri-lesional vasogenic oedema and control neurologic symptoms in the short-term. It is suspected that high-dose corticosteroids prevent immune activation and attenuate the benefit of immune checkpoint blockade.

The blood brain barrier comprises of endothelial cells, astrocytes and pericytes. Usually the passage of molecules from blood to the brain parenchyma is limited under physiological conditions [7]. However, research has shown that activated T-cells can cross the blood–brain barrier - raising the possibility of treatment using immunotherapy [8]. The endothelial cells of the blood brain barrier in brain metastases are thought to be able to initiate an inflammatory cascade that activates immune cells [9]. Berghoff et al. have shown, using immunohistochemical analysis of melanoma brain metastases, that three-quarters of these lesions exhibit CD3+ tumour-infiltrating-lymphocytes and tumour cells were PD-1 positive in half of cases [10] (**Table 1**).

In contrast to carcinomas, such as breast and lung, melanoma brain metastases display a diffuse lymphocytic infiltrate throughout the tumour mass as opposed to a stromal infiltrate [11]. These pathologic data provide strong evidence that adaptive immune responses can be active in the distinct microenvironment of the brain.

Lepto-meningeal metastases are a deadly and feared complication of malignant melanoma and also occur commonly in breast and lung cancers. They are common in haematological malignancy but much rarer in solid tumours where they usually manifest in the presence of advanced metastatic disease in multiple organ systems. Lepto-meningeal metastasis, also sometimes known as neoplastic meningitis, occurs when cancer cells disseminate to the arachnoid and/or pia mater covering the central nervous systemic tissue in the brain and/or spinal cord. They typically cause rapidly-progressive, and often fatal, neurological deficits due to infiltration of cranial nerves, spinal cord and nerve root compression (radiculopathy), symptoms of meningitis and raised intracranial pressure. Treatment is usually supportive and there is very little evidence for any anti-cancer treatment being effective although intra-thecal chemotherapy has been used as has cranio-spinal radiotherapy which is poorly tolerated in adults.

The vast majority of clinical trials for metastatic melanoma exclude patients with brain metastases, and certainly those with symptomatic lesions. Therefore, there is a paucity of clinical evidence to guide decision making in terms of therapeutic options for this patient population. The current clinical evidence base comprises small, retrospective studies. The majority of patients with metastatic melanoma will develop brain or lepto-meningeal metastases at some point in their disease trajectory [12], therefore this chapter will provide a good summary to help clinicians to understand and manage this group of patients.

Drug	Target	FDA approval date	Treatment schedule
Ipilimumab	CTLA-4	March 2011	3 mg/kg administered intravenously every 3 weeks
Pembrolizumab	PD-1	December 2014	2 mg/kg administered intravenously every 3 weeks or 200 mg every 3 weeks/400 mg every 6 weeks
Nivolumab	PD-1	September 2014	3 mg/kg administered intravenously every 2 weeks or 240 mg every 2 weeks/480 mg every 4 weeks

Table 1.
Immunotherapy and treatment schedule.

2. Immune checkpoint inhibitors for metastatic melanoma

The therapeutic options for patients with metastatic melanoma, previously restricted to dacarbazine chemotherapy (DTIC, alkylating agent) [13] and immunotherapy with high-dose intravenous interleukin-2 [14], have expanded to include immune checkpoint inhibitors and BRAF targeted therapy in recent times and the outlook has become somewhat less guarded with long-term survival being achieved in a proportion of patients. Importantly, in terms of randomised, comparative large-scale clinical trials no such evidence exists for DTIC or IL-2 despite FDA approval in 1975 and 1998 respectively. Immune checkpoint inhibitors are monoclonal antibodies that disrupt the CTLA-4/CD28 and PD-1/PD-L1 interactions, and by so doing, lead to improvements in T-cell priming by dendritic cells and cytotoxic T-cell effector function respectively. These treatments, such as ipilimumab (anti CTLA-4) and pembrolizumab (anti-PD-1), attenuate T-cell inhibitory signals and generate enhanced, sustained and powerful anti-melanoma immune responses that can be associated with durable disease control. It is noteworthy that the first systemic therapy proven to confer a survival advantage in metastatic melanoma was the anti CTLA-4 antibody ipilimumab and this was the first time in a randomised clinical trial that an increase in overall survival had been achieved in this disease [15]. The comparator group in this trial was treatment with an HLA-A2 restricted gp100 peptide vaccine not placebo and patients had received prior chemotherapy or IL-2. Toxicities of ipilimumab can be severe and unpredictable and in the pivotal study, the treatment-related death rate was 2.1% although this has diminished over time as physicians' experience and patient education improves. However, with ipilimumab monotherapy only approximately one in five patients achieve long-term overall survival and patients with high volume metastatic disease, elevated serum lactate dehydrogenase levels, low serum albumen, rapidly progressive course and brain metastases seldom derive benefit benefit [16]. In previously untreated metastatic melanoma patients, high-dose ipilimumab monotherapy (10 mg/kg) in combination with dacarbazine chemotherapy outperformed chemotherapy in terms of overall and progression-free survival and to a lesser extent objective response rate [17]. From the clinical perspective, the United Kingdom [18] National Institute for Health and Care Excellence (NICE) approved Ipilimumab for the treatment of metastatic melanoma in 2012 [19], followed by Pembrolizumab and Nivolumab that target the PD-1 axis in 2015. Combination immunotherapy with concurrent ipilimumab and nivolumab has also been available since 2017 for the treatment of metastatic melanoma with favourable outcome compared to ipilimumab monotherapy. This clinical trial was, however, not sufficiently powered to definitively determine if combination immunotherapy was superior to nivolumab monotherapy [20]. Ipilimumab and nivolumab can achieve objective radiologic responses rates of approximately 60% and the likelihood of 5-year overall survival is 53%. These agents, especially anti PD-1 monotherapy, are better tolerated than chemotherapy [21], and demonstrated a better progression-free survival outcome with lower toxicities [22].

In a randomised Phase II clinical trial, patients with ipilimumab and targeted therapy (if BRAF mutant) refractory advanced melanoma had improved progression-free survival when treated with pembrolizumab compared with investigators choice of cytotoxic chemotherapy with a likelihood of 6-month progression-free survival of 34% versus 16%. Serious treatment-related adverse events were far less common with immunotherapy – 11% versus 26% with chemotherapy. The likelihood of radiologic response was 5 times higher with pembrolizumab (21%) than chemotherapy (4%) [23].

Selection of patients who are most likely to benefit from immune checkpoint blockade remains largely an elusive goal, although potential biomarkers are emerging and these include a high somatic mutational burden with resultant abundant neo-epitopes for immune recognition [24], a greater diversity within the faecal microbiome and the presence therein of specific bacterial species [25], the level of PD-L1 expression on tumour cells and tumour-associated leukocytes [26] and density of CD8 T-cell tumoural infiltrate [27]. Identification of predictive biomarkers for immunotherapy would allow futile treatment and associated toxicities to be avoided in patients unlikely to benefit.

Ipilimumab was the first checkpoint inhibitor to be used in patients with CNS metastases. In 2012, Margolin et al. published a phase 2 study involving 72 melanoma patients with CNS metastases who received intravenous ipilimumab. Intra-cranial disease control (defined as objective response or stable disease for at least 3 months) was achieved in 24% of the patients who were asymptomatic and not receiving corticosteroids and 10% in those with symptomatic, steroid-requiring lesions [28]. However, in a real-world study of ipilimumab for metastatic melanoma patients in the UK, median overall survival for those with brain metastases was 3.5 months [16]. This was followed by another open-label phase 2 trial using intravenous Pembrolizumab [29]. Of 18 patients enrolled into that study, 22% achieved disease control intracranially. Recently, Tawbi et al. published in the New England Journal of Medicine a larger trial involving 94 patients being treated with combination immunotherapy [30]. In patients with small (less than 3 cm) asymptomatic brain metastases, the intracranial clinical benefit rate (objective response or stable disease for at least 6 months) was 57%, there were also higher chances of grade 3 and 4 toxicities (55%). The rate of radiologic complete response within the brain is notable at 26% and this may be a surrogate marker of long-term survival. Intra-cranial responses were achieved rapidly with a median time to response of 2.3 months. The rate of intra-cranial response was in fact slightly numerically higher than that of extra-cranial metastases. Similar findings were noted in Long's study including patients with lesion size up to 40 mm with an intra-cranial response rate of 46% (in pre-treated patients) and 56% in systemic-therapy naïve patients and 53% of patients were free of intra-cranial progression at 6 months, using ipilimumab and nivolumab. However, combination immunotherapy was of marginal benefit in patients with progression after prior local treatment for brain metastases, neurologic symptoms or lepto-meningeal disease with a single partial intra-cranial response amongst 16 patients, only 13% were free of intra-cranial progression at 6 months and median overall survival was poor at 5.1 months (similar to that of historic patients treated with supportive care with or without whole brain radiotherapy) [31]. Ipilimumab monotherapy, even at doses as high as 10 mg/kg with associated toxicities, was also ineffective in patients with neurologic symptoms with an intra-cranial response rate of 5% and median overall survival of 3.7 months as described by Margolin et al. [28] Anti PD-1 monotherapy appears to be a valid treatment option with intra-cranial response rates of 22–26% and median overall survival of 18 months [32]. However, the durability of responses when patients have brain metastases remains uncertain, and by way of comparison, median overall survival for patients without brain metastases treated with pembrolizumab was 24 months and 38.6 months in treatment-naive patients [33].

When taken as a whole, most clinical trials of immunotherapy appear to show potential clinical benefit to melanoma patients with CNS metastases, with combination immunotherapy possibly providing the best clinical outcomes but at the cost of higher toxicity.

3. Targeted therapy for intracranial metastatic melanoma

Approximately 45 to 50% of patients with metastatic cutaneous melanoma harbour missense mutations involving the BRAF proto-oncogene (codon 600) and in these patients MAP kinase targeted therapies such dabrafenib with trametinib or encorafenib with binimetinib are a valid treatment option with high rates of radiologic response including intra-cranial responses. There is no randomised clinical trial evidence to guide the selection of 1st line systemic therapy in BRAF mutant patients, concurrent treatment with MAP kinase inhibitors and immune checkpoint inhibitors remains a highly experimental approach albeit with some early signals that combination treatment can be safely delivered and there is no clinically useful predictive biomarker for immunotherapy benefit. This remains a nuanced clinical dilemma for the oncologist and patient. RAF and MEK inhibitors have direct anti-proliferative effects on the melanoma cells and do not rely on using the immune system as an effector and their effectiveness is not blunted by immunosuppressive therapies such as corticosteroids. Therefore, many patients with melanoma brain metastasis have received targeted therapy in the first line setting with rapid tumour control and neurological improvement in the majority but durability of response is limited with typical intra-cranial progression free survival of 6–8 months. Rapid progression of metastatic disease, and particularly CNS metastases, when refractoriness to RAF and MEK inhibitors inevitably develops often leads to a sharp decline in performance status and many patients are unable to receive or benefit from immunotherapeutic approaches in the second line setting. In fact, an Australian retrospective study found that only 35% of patients discontinuing front-line targeted therapy for progressive disease went on to receive subsequent lines of systemic therapy [34]. There is also biological evidence that the increased melanoma differentiation antigen expression, enhanced dendritic cell function and increased CD8 T-cell infiltration driven by RAF–MEK inhibitors early on in treatment (2 weeks) is lost at the time of tumour progression, creating an 'immune desert' environmental that is hostile to the effects of immune checkpoint inhibitors. Therefore, where small asymptomatic brain metastases are present or when brain lesions have been treated with ablative radiotherapy, immunotherapy should be the preferred initial treatment.

4. Whole brain radiotherapy and stereotactic radiosurgery for intracranial metastatic melanoma

Radiotherapy is widely used to treat intracranial melanoma, i.e., brain metastasis, in order to control disease, alleviate symptoms and even improve survival. The two main forms of radiotherapy are stereotactic radiosurgery (SRS) and whole brain radiotherapy (WBRT). Radiotherapy planning, dose and schedule, and outcomes differs between SRS and WBRT.

4.1 Whole brain radiotherapy

As the name implies WBRT involves the irradiation of the entire intracranial contents, tumour and normal brain tissue alike. WBRT is often used when intracranial disease is extensive, such as large and/or multiple brain metastasis or leptomeningeal disease, and when radical treatment is not possible. Even with WBRT, overall survival is poor in the order of 6 months and patients are unlikely to survive long enough to develop late toxicity of irradiation of normal brain such as neurocognitive impairment. Treatment set up typically involves a pair of opposing photon beams, from the patients left and right, which converge in the mid-plane to deliver dose throughout the cranium. 20Gy in five daily fractions and 30Gy in ten fractions over two weeks are two commonly used conventional WBRT schedules worldwide with the latter the standard schedule in the United Kingdom [35]. Clinical trials did not demonstrate any benefit in improvement of neurological function or overall survival with dose escalation over conventional WBRT [36]. Despite widespread use worldwide over decades, only two clinical trials compared WBRT with best supportive care. The first, published in 1971, reported no difference in survival between WBRT and oral prednisolone alone but the study was conducted in the pre computed tomography era and hampered by a small cohort and inadequate statistics [37]. The QUARTZ trial reported in 2016 is a multi-centred, statistically powered trial conducted on patients with non-small cell lung cancer (NSCLC) with brain metastases unsuitable for radical treatment. There was no significant difference in overall survival and quality of life between patients treated with WBRT compared to dexamethasone and best supportive care alone. Overall survival was in the order of 9 weeks which is a reflection of poor prognosis with brain metastases and the limited effect of WBRT. Subgroup analysis indicated that patients under 60 or with five of more brain metastases might derive a survival benefit from WBRT [38]. Although this trial was limited to NSCLC, it is likely that similar results will be observed with WBRT to brain metastases from other cancer types. WBRT is no longer default option in managing brain metastases unsuitable for radical treatment given the lack of clear benefit in survival or quality of life, potential toxicity and inconvenience to the patient. Instead, the clinician should consider patient factors, such as age, performance status, systemic disease status and patient wishes, in tailoring a patient-centred management plan which includes best supportive care.

4.2 Stereotactic radiosurgery

Patients with limited brain metastases such as solitary or oligometastatic metastases or small volume disease, could benefit from treatment such as neurosurgery and SRS which are more targeted and radical than WBRT. These treatment modalities can achieve superior long-term control compared to WBRT. For instance, local control rate after SRS is in the order of 70–90% at 1 year [3, 39–42]. Decision to treat with SRS or neurosurgery should be made in a multi-disciplinary setting. A brain metastasis that is solitary, accessible, or large volume causing pressure symptoms is an ideal candidate for neurosurgery whereas lesions that are small in volume, surgically inaccessible or multiple are suitable for SRS. Patient factors such as surgical and anaesthetic risk and comorbidities need to be taken into account too [43]. Outcomes after neurosurgery and SRS are similar; a meta-analysis reported non-significant difference in local control between SRS and neurosurgery at 1 year, and non-significant difference in overall survival at 1 and 2 years [44].

Unlike WBRT, SRS is focused high dose radiotherapy on the brain metastases with steep dose fall off to reduce irradiation of normal brain. Multiple brain metastases up to a total of 20 ml can be treated. The volume limit is intended to limit collateral dose to normal brain. Treatment set up involves the patients being immobilised either with a stereotactic frame or custom-made thermoplastic mask which serve to minimise movement and error during treatment delivery. Small lesions such as those under

2 cm can be treated with 20 Gy in a single fraction while larger lesions or those close to critical structures such as the brain stem or optic chiasm are treated with lower dose of 15–18 Gy in a single fraction or a fractionated schedule such as 27Gy in three fractions. Acute toxicities of SRS include headache, nausea, fatigue and risk of seizure and are often self-limiting and managed with steroids.

The addition of WBRT to SRS reduces the risk of intracranial recurrence but this does not translate into a survival benefit [3, 42, 45]. Intracranial recurrence, either with local recurrence of previously treated lesion or distant recurrence of new lesions, can potentially be treated with repeat SRS which obviates the need for upfront WBRT. WBRT also increases the risk of late neurotoxicity such as leukoencephalopathy and neurocognitive impairment which can manifest many months after treatment and result in significant detriment in quality of life and function [42, 45, 46]. Late neurotoxicity is a significant concern especially for patients who will otherwise have long term systemic disease control, such as patients with melanoma with good response to immunotherapy. The addition of WBRT to SRS is therefore not the standard of care in the United Kingdom. Instead, radiological surveillance with MRI to detect recurrence is performed after SRS [10].

4.3 Radiotherapy and immunotherapy

Radiotherapy can disrupt the blood–brain barrier allowing the entry of drugs into the central nervous system circulation. Concurrent radiotherapy and immunotherapy might have a synergistic effect stimulating the immune response resulting in greater anti-cancer effect. Several retrospective studies have reported excellent outcomes with concurrent radiotherapy and immunotherapy for melanoma. One study on reported overall survival of 56 months with SRS and immunotherapy compared to 24 months and 14 months with immunotherapy alone and SRS alone respectively, while another study reported significantly longer overall survival (15.9 months vs. 6.1 months) and lower cumulative incidence of neurologic death (9% vs. 23%) with SRS and immunotherapy compared to SRS alone [47, 48]. The synergistic effect of radiotherapy and immunotherapy on the immune response in theory could result in more severe acute toxicity, however these studies also report good safety profile with low incidences of grade III or greater toxicity. Treatment scheduling and long-term outcomes and toxicities of combined immunotherapy and radiotherapy are areas of ongoing research interest.

5. Conclusions

The landscape of systemic treatments of MBM patients has undergone tremendous evolution over the past decades and there has been major improvement in outcome for this disease.

Immunotherapy is a relatively safe option for MBM patients with anti-PD-1 having least toxicity and associated with no reported treatment related death. On the other hand, Ipilimumab is associated with increase in immune related toxicities but Ipilimumab and Nivolumab has shown increase in overall survival when comparing with monotherapy. Also, combination with radiotherapy and immunotherapy provides a higher response rate but potential increase in CNS toxicities. More studies are needed to determine the progression free survival, patient's satisfaction and quality of life as well as assessing the cost effectiveness of the treatments.

Combination of immunotherapy with cytotoxic chemotherapy or targeted therapy may also be a potential therapeutic approach, but further understanding of drug mechanism is required.

Acknowledgements

Special thanks to Professor Poulam Patel and Dr. Ankit Rao for their ongoing encouragement and guidance.

Conflict of interest

The authors declare no conflict of interest.

Author details

Hiu Kwan Carolyn Tang* and Joon Wee Ho
Nottingham City Hospital, Nottingham, UK

*Address all correspondence to: ht8000@my.bristol.ac.uk

References

[1] Davies MA, Liu P, McIntyre S, Kim KB, Papadopoulos N, Hwu WJ, et al. Prognostic factors for survival in melanoma patients with brain metastases. Cancer. 2011;**117**(8): 1687-1696

[2] Lorigan JG, Wallace S, Mavligit GM. The prevalence and location of metastases from ocular melanoma: Imaging study in 110 patients. AJR. American Journal of Roentgenology. 1991;**157**(6):1279-1281

[3] Brown PD, Brown CA, Pollock BE, Gorman DA, Foote RL. Stereotactic radiosurgery for patients with "radioresistant" brain metastases. Neurosurgery. 2002;**51**(3):656-665 discussion 65-7

[4] Reynders K, Illidge T, Siva S, Chang JY, De Ruysscher D. The abscopal effect of local radiotherapy: Using immunotherapy to make a rare event clinically relevant. Cancer Treatment Reviews. 2015;**41**(6):503-510

[5] Frey Benjamin RY, Lorenz K. Antitumor immune responses induced by ionizing irradiation and further immune stimulation. Cancer Immunology, Immunotherapy. 2013;**63**(1):29-36

[6] Twyman-Saint Victor C, Rech AJ, Maity A, Rengan R, Pauken KE, Stelekati E, et al. Radiation and dual checkpoint blockade activate non-redundant immune mechanisms in cancer. Nature. 2015;**520**(7547):373-377

[7] Carson MJ, Doose JM, Melchior B, Schmid CD, Ploix CC. CNS immune privilege: Hiding in plain sight. Immunological Reviews. 2006;**213**:48-65

[8] Wilson EH, Weninger W, Hunter CA. Trafficking of immune cells in the central nervous system. The Journal of Clinical Investigation. 2010;**120**:1368-1379

[9] Hamilton A, Sibson NR. Role of the systemic immune system in brain metastasis. Molecular and Cellular Neurosciences. 2013;**53**:42-51

[10] Berghoff AS, Ricken G, Widhalm G, Rajky O, Dieckmann K, Birner P, et al. Tumour-infiltrating lymphocytes and expression of programmed death ligand 1 (PD-L1) in melanoma brain metastases. Histopathology. 2015;**66**(2):289-299

[11] Harter PN, Bernatz S, Scholz A, Zeiner PS, Zinke J, Kiyose M, et al. Distribution and prognostic relevance of tumor-infiltrating lymphocytes (TILs) and PD-1/PD-L1 immune checkpoints in human brain metastases. Oncotarget. 2015;**6**(38):40836-40849

[12] Bafaloukos D, Gogas H. The treatment of brain metastases in melanoma patients. Cancer Treatment Reviews. 2004;**30**(6):515-520

[13] Chapman PB, Einhorn LH, Meyers ML, Saxman S, Destro AN, Panageas KS, et al. Phase III multicenter randomized trial of the Dartmouth regimen versus dacarbazine in patients with metastatic melanoma. Journal of Clinical Oncology. 1999;**17**(9):2745-2751

[14] Atkins MB, Lotze MT, Dutcher JP, Fisher RI, Weiss G, Margolin K, et al. High-dose recombinant interleukin 2 therapy for patients with metastatic melanoma: Analysis of 270 patients treated between 1985 and 1993. Journal of Clinical Oncology. 1999;**17**(7):2105-2116

[15] Hodi FS, O'Day SJ, McDermott DF, Weber RW, Sosman JA, Haanen JB,

et al. Improved survival with Ipilimumab in patients with metastatic melanoma. The New England Journal of Medicine. 2010;**363**(8):711-723. DOI: 10.1056/NEJMoa1003466

[16] Ahmad SS, Qian W, Ellis S, Mason E, Khattak MA, Gupta A, et al. Ipilimumab in the real world: The UK expanded access programme experience in previously treated advanced melanoma patients. Melanoma Research. 2015;**25**(5):432-442

[17] Robert C, Thomas L, Bondarenko I, O'Day S, Weber J, Garbe C, et al. Ipilimumab plus Dacarbazine for previously untreated metastatic melanoma. The New England Journal of Medicine. 2011;**364**:2517-2526. DOI: 10.1056/NEJMoa1104621

[18] Wei S, C. Fundamental mechanisms of immune checkpoint blockade therapy. Cancer Discovery. 2019;**8**(9):1069-1086

[19] NICE. Ipilimumab for Previously Treated Advanced (Unresectable or Metastatic) Melanoma. Guidance and Guidelines. United Kingdom: NICE; 2012 Available from: https://www.nice.org.uk/guidance/ta268/chapter/1-Guidance

[20] Wolchok JD, Chiarion-Sileni V, Gonzalez R, Rutkowski P, Grob J-J, Cowey CL, et al. Overall survival with combined Nivolumab and Ipilimumab in advanced melanoma. The New England Journal of Medicine. 2017;**377**:1345-1356. DOI: 10.1056/NEJMoa1709684

[21] Nishijima TF, Shachar SS, Nyrop KA, Muss HB. Safety and tolerability of PD-1/PD-L1 inhibitors compared with chemotherapy in patients with advanced cancer: A meta-analysis. The Oncologist. 2017;**22**(4):470-479

[22] Larkin J, Chiarion-Sileni V, Gonzalez R, Grob JJ, Cowey CL, Lao CD, et al. Combined Nivolumab and Ipilimumab or monotherapy in untreated melanoma. The New England Journal of Medicine. 2015;**373**(1):23-34

[23] Ribas A, Puzanov I, Dummer R, Schadendorf D, Hamid O, Robert C, et al. Pembrolizumab versus investigator-choice chemotherapy for ipilimumab-refractory melanoma (KEYNOTE-002): A randomised, controlled, phase 2 trial. The Lancet Oncology. 2015;**16**(8):908-918

[24] Snyder A, Makarov V, Merghoub T, Yuan J, Zaretsky JM, Desrichard A, et al. Genetic basis for clinical response to CTLA-4 blockade in melanoma. The New England Journal of Medicine. 2014, 2014;**371**(23):2189-2199. DOI: 10.1056/NEJMoa1406498

[25] Gopalakrishnan V, Spencer CN, Nezi L, Reuben A, Andrews MC, Karpinets TV, et al. Gut microbiome modulates response to anti-PD-1 immunotherapy in melanoma patients. Science. 2018;**359**(6371):97-103

[26] Daud AI, Wolchok JD, Robert C, Hwu WJ, Weber JS, Ribas A, et al. Programmed death-ligand 1 expression and response to the anti-programmed death 1 antibody Pembrolizumab in melanoma. Journal of Clinical Oncology. 2016;**34**(34):4102-4109

[27] Tumeh PC, Harview CL, Yearley JH, Shintaku IP, Taylor EJ, Robert L, et al. PD-1 blockade induces responses by inhibiting adaptive immune resistance. Nature. 2014;**515**(7528):568-571

[28] Margolin K, Ernstoff MS, Hamid O, Lawrence D, McDermott D, Puzanov I, et al. Ipilimumab in patients with melanoma and brain metastases: An open-label, phase 2 trial. The Lancet Oncology. 2012;**13**(5):459-465

[29] Goldberg SB, Gettinger SN, Mahajan A, Chiang AC, Herbst RS, Sznol M, et al. Pembrolizumab for patients with melanoma or non-small-cell lung cancer and untreated brain metastases: Early analysis of a non-randomised, open-label, phase 2 trial. The Lancet Oncology. 2016;**17**(7):976-983

[30] Tawbi HA, Forsyth PA, Algazi A, Hamid O, Hodi FS, Moschos SJ, et al. Combined Nivolumab and Ipilimumab in melanoma metastatic to the brain. The New England Journal of Medicine. 2018;**379**:722-730. DOI: 10.1056/NEJMoa1805453

[31] Long GV, Atkinson V, Lo S, Sandhu S, Guminski AD, Brown MP, et al. Combination nivolumab and ipilimumab or nivolumab alone in melanoma brain metastases: A multicentre randomised phase 2 study. The Lancet Oncology. 2018;**19**(5):672-681

[32] Kluger HM, Chiang V, Mahajan A, Zito CR, Sznol M, Tran T, et al. Long-term survival of patients with melanoma with active brain metastases treated with Pembrolizumab on a phase II trial. Journal of Clinical Oncology. 2019;**37**(1):52-60

[33] Hamid O, Robert C, Daud A, Hodi FS, Hwu WJ, Kefford R, et al. Five-year survival outcomes for patients with advanced melanoma treated with pembrolizumab in KEYNOTE-001. Annals of Oncology. 2019;**30**(4):582-588

[34] Ackerman A, Klein O, McDermott DF, Wang W, Ibrahim N, Lawrence DP, et al. Outcomes of patients with metastatic melanoma treated with immunotherapy prior to or after BRAF inhibitors. Cancer. 2014;**120**(11):1695-1701

[35] The Royal College of Radiologists. Radiotherapy Dose Fractionation. Third ed. The Royal College of Radiologists, United Kingdom; 2019. Available online: https://www.rcr.ac.uk/system/files/publication/field_publication_files/bfco163_dose_fractionation_2nd_ed_march2017.pdf

[36] Mn T, Xu W, Rks W, et al. Whole brain radiotherapy for the treatment of newly diagnosed multiple brain metastases. Cochrane Database of Systematic Reviews. 2012;**4**:CD003869. DOI: 10.1002/14651858.CD003869

[37] Horton J, Baxter D, Olson K. The management of metastases to the brain by irradiation and corticosteroids. The American Journal of Roentgenology, Radium Therapy, and Nuclear Medicine. 1971;**111**:334-336

[38] Mulvenna P, Nankivell M, Barton R, et al. Dexamethasone and supportive care with or without whole brain radiotherapy in treating patients with non-small cell lung cancer with brain metastases unsuitable for resection or stereotactic radiotherapy (QUARTZ): Results from a phase 3, non-inferiority. Lancet. 2016;**388**(10055):2004-2014. DOI: 10.1016/S0140-6736(16)30825-X

[39] Auchter RM, Lamond JP, Alexander E, et al. A multiinstitutional outcome and prognostic factor analysis of radiosurgery for resectable single brain metastasis. International Journal of Radiation Oncology, Biology, Physics. 1996;**35**(1):27-35. DOI: 10.1016/S0360-3016(96)85008-5

[40] Sneed PK, Suh JH, Goetsch SJ, et al. A multi-institutional review of radiosurgery alone vs. radiosurgery with whole brain radiotherapy as the initial management of brain metastases. International Journal of Radiation Oncology, Biology, Physics.

2002;**53**(3):519-526. DOI: 10.1016/S0360-3016(02)02770-0

[41] Kondziolka D, Patel A, Lunsford LD, Kassam A, Flickinger JC. Stereotactic radiosurgery plus whole brain radiotherapy versus radiotherapy alone for patients with multiple brain metastases. International Journal of Radiation Oncology. 1999;**45**(2):427-434. DOI: 10.1016/S0360-3016(99)00198-4

[42] Chang EL, Wefel JS, Hess KR, et al. Neurocognition in patients with brain metastases treated with radiosurgery or radiosurgery plus whole-brain irradiation: A randomised controlled trial. The Lancet Oncology. 2009;**10**(11):1037-1044. DOI: 10.1016/S1470-2045(09)70263-3

[43] NICE guidelines [NG99]. Brain Tumours (Primary) and Brain Metastases in over 16s. Guidance NICE. The National Institute for Health and Care Excellence (NICE), United Kingdom; 2021. Available online: https://www.nice.org.uk/guidance/ng99/chapter/recommendations#follow-up-for-glioma

[44] Krist D, Naik A, Thompson C, Kwok S, Janbahan M, Olivero W, et al. Management of brain metastasis. Surgical resection versus stereotactic radiotherapy: A meta-analysis. Neuro-Oncology Advances. 2022;**4**. DOI: 10.1093/noajnl/vdac033

[45] Aoyama H, Tago M, Kato N, et al. Neurocognitive function of patients with brain metastasis who received either whole brain radiotherapy plus stereotactic radiosurgery or radiosurgery alone. International Journal of Radiation Oncology, Biology, Physics. 2007;**68**(5):1388-1395. DOI: 10.1016/j.ijrobp.2007.03.048

[46] Monaco EA, Faraji AH, Berkowitz O, et al. Leukoencephalopathy after whole-brain radiation therapy plus radiosurgery versus radiosurgery alone for metastatic lung cancer. Cancer. 2013;**119**(1):226-232. DOI: 10.1002/cncr.27504

[47] O'Shea PJ, Tatineni V, Rauf Y, et al. Outcomes of immunotherapy (ICI) alone vs. stereotactic radiosurgery (SRS) alone vs. ICI and SRS combined in melanoma brain metastasis. International Journal of Radiation Oncology. 2021;**111**(3):e575-e576. DOI: 10.1016/j.ijrobp.2021.07.1550

[48] Lanier CM, Hughes R, Ahmed T, et al. Immunotherapy is associated with improved survival and decreased neurologic death after SRS for brain metastases from lung and melanoma primaries. Neuro-Oncology Practice. 2019;**6**(5):402-409. DOI: 10.1093/nop/npz004

Section 7

Novel Therapies for Advanced Disease

Chapter 9

Novel Therapies in Clinical Development for Advanced Disease

Álvaro Sánchez Arráez, Sonia Maciá and Eduardo Castañón

Abstract

Recent advances in melanoma treatment have supposed a dramatic transformation overcoming the situation that was faced 15 years ago, when advanced melanoma was a fatal disease, with less than five percent of patients being alive after 1 year of diagnosis. However, in spite of the impressive improvement that has been achieved with immunotherapies and targeted therapies that are completely part of the standard landscape for treatment, additional therapeutic advances are still needed. In this chapter, we review those systemic and local treatments which are undergoing clinical development, explaining their mechanisms of action and the already presented either preliminary or final results, most of them in terms of response rate.

Keywords: immunotherapy, targeted therapy, intratumoral, citokines, oncolytic virus, Pattern recognition receptor, new therapeutic targets

1. Introduction

The treatment of metastatic melanoma has evolved dramatically in the past recent years, provoking an important paradigm shift [1], with huge progress in melanoma survival. The development of targeted therapies such as BRAF and MEK 2–6 inhibitors [2–6], as well as the appearance of different molecules targeting program death 1 (PD1) [7, 8] and anti-cytotoxic T-lymphocyte associated antigen (CTLA4) [9–11], has contributed to improving the prognosis of metastatic melanoma, turning melanoma to one of the most responsive tumors to these kinds of therapies.

However, there is still a high percentage of patients who do not respond to first-line immunotherapy. Besides, those patients with *B-RAF* mutant disease who develop progression after both targeted therapy and immunotherapy (regardless of the order of use) face a poor prognosis. Hence, in these two groups of patients, being both considered as patients developing progression to immunotherapy, the disease is still considered an important medical need. Hence, the development of new potential therapies is key, and extensive clinical research is ongoing to develop new treatments which may improve prognosis in all patients.

2. Citokines

a. Interleukin-2 (IL-2)

Interleukin 2 is a cytokine that promotes the growth and expansion of T lymphocytes and NK cells [12]. Its antitumor activity has been tested in patients with renal carcinoma and patients with melanoma [13]. However, its toxicity profile (hypotension, capillary leak syndrome...) prevents it from being a standard of care. To try to reduce the toxicity associated with IL2, different strategies have been designed. One of the most developed molecules is Bempegaldesleukin (BEMPEG) [14]. BEMPEG is a pegylated molecule, thereby reducing systemic IL2 exposure. In addition, it has a higher affinity for the IL2 receptor subunit CD122, thereby decreasing the activation of the IL2 pathway that is associated with most serious side effects. However, despite promising results in melanoma patients in the PIVOT-02 [15] study, no increased benefit of BEMPE in combination with Nivolumab versus Nivolumab alone was seen in first-line metastatic melanoma setting (PIVOT IO-001) [16].

b. Interleukin 12 (IL-12)

Interleukin 12 is a cytokine mainly produced by monocytes [17]. It is one of the most important stimuli for the activation of NK cells.

In recent years, the role of systemic and intratumoral administration of recombinant IL12 has been studied in different settings [18]. Recently, a new formulation consisting of an IL12 coding plasmid (Tavokinogene telseplasmid or TAVO) has been shown to achieve a sustained concentration of cytokines in the tumor microenvironment [19]. In 2014, data from the OMS100 trial were presented [20]. The results were encouraging in patients with metastatic melanoma with injectable lesions who were exposed to TAVO in combination with electroporation. This study showed a significant response rate and interestingly, cases of maintained responses over time. Years later, very promising data was presented showing that combination of TAVO and Pembrolizumab in patients with metastatic melanoma may be an optimal approach [21].

The phase III KEYNOTE-C87 trial promises interesting results as it evaluates the role of TAVO in combination with Pembrolizumab vs. standard treatment in patients with metastatic melanoma who have already been exposed to prior immunotherapy.

c. Transforming growth factor beta (TGF-beta)

Transforming growth factor beta is a cytokine with different roles involved in vascular diseases, autoimmune diseases, and carcinogenesis [22]. It seems that the effect of TGF beta could be dual since it has both tumor suppressor and pro-inflammatory activity, favoring invasiveness and capacity for metastasis [23].

Different formulations are being tested, such as SHR-1701, which has two targets, PD1 receptor ligand (PDL1) and the receptor II of TGF beta [24]. SHR-1701 is under evaluation in combination with Temozolomide for patients with metastatic melanoma (NCT05106023).

Another formulation currently under evaluation is Vactocertib, an oral inhibitor of the serine/threonine kinase TGFBR1 [25]. Its efficacy is currently being tested in combination with Pembrolizumab in patients with metastatic melanoma.

3. Oncolytic viruses

Oncolytic viruses constitute a very interesting therapeutic weapon since usually they have the capacity to infect only tumor cells, causing them to lyse, and hardly affecting normal cells [26]. Currently, there are different formulations, from viruses with exclusively oncolytic capacity to viruses with the ability to use the machinery of the infected cell to produce different immune stimulators.

Among the most developed viruses already approved, we find Talimogene laherparepvec (T-VEC) [27]. T-VEC is a herpes family virus that is capable of producing GM-CSF. T-VEC provokes not only cellular lysis but also increases the concentration of GM-CSF, thus, favoring a cellular enrichment by dendritic cells and cytotoxic T lymphocytes in the tumor niche. The first results of the OPTIM trial for patients with metastatic melanoma were presented in 2015 and led to TVEC approval by FDA27. Later, it was observed that T-VEC infection could increase the expression of PD1 in the tumor bed, so an attempt was made to show whether adding Pembrolizumab could improve the results of T-VEC injection [28]. However, the phase III study that sought to answer this question was not significant [29]. There are other viruses that have shown efficacy for the treatment of metastatic melanoma, such as the TILT-123 [30] adenovirus (with the ability to produce cytokines such as TNF alpha and IL12), the PVSRIPO 31 virus [31] (a modification of the polio vaccine), Oncos-10232 [32] (adenovirus producing GM-CSF), CAVATAK [33] (enterovirus with oncolytic capacity) or Ad-RTS-hIL-1233 [34] (adenovirus producing IL-12).

4. Intratumoral therapies

One of the greatest advances in immunotherapy is the possibility of intratumoral administration [35]. Although the intratumoral route has been known since the beginning of the 20th century, there are currently many clinical trials using this route [36]. Theoretically, the intratumoral route would allow to use of lower doses of the different agents, obtain a pharmacodynamic profile in real-time, as well as facilitate the combination with different drugs, since a much more manageable toxicity profile is usually seen. In addition, intratumoral therapy has an effect at distant non-injected metastatic sites, in what we know as *abscopal effect* (if the therapy is purely intratumoral) or an anesthetic effect (if the intratumoral strategy is combined with the intravenous one). Currently, there are available results from different molecules administered intratumorally. However, as of today, most positive results from phase II trials with intratumoral agents have not been confirmed in subsequent phase III studies. Interestingly, very positive data in terms of response rates have been seen in the early phases of trials. These therapies face important challenges, starting with the selection of suitable patients, the assessment of response, and the injection procedure *per se,* which may require the involvement of different departments, such as interventional radiology or surgery. Trials with these kind of agents are very heterogeneous, and characteristics of patients are extremely different among different studies; besides, primary endpoints also differ. Looking retrospectively at the data, it seems that those patients with only cutaneous-subcutaneous disease, achieve the highest benefit, but positive preliminary data have been seen also in mucosal melanoma and overall population, with response rates over 25% in the second line setting, as presented below.

4.1 Pattern recognition receptor (PRR) agonists

Within the PRRs agonists, various molecules have been tested in patients with metastatic melanoma.

a. **TLR9 agonists**

TLR9 is present in the endosome of myeloid cells, B lymphocytes, and dendritic cells [37]. Its functions, although varied, facilitate a pro-inflammatory state in the tumor niche. To date, different intratumoral TLR9 agonists have been tested in patients with metastatic melanoma. Many of them have had negative results, although many others show some signs of activity. CMP-001 has been tested in different scenarios, alone and in combination with an antiPD1 agent [38], not only in patients with metastatic melanoma but also in patients with high-risk locally advanced melanoma in the neoadjuvant setting [39].
On the other hand, the results of the SINERGY-001 trial should be highlighted, which investigated the role of TLR9 agonist SD-101 in combination with Pembrolizumab in patients diagnosed with metastatic melanoma who had previously been treated with antiPD1 [40]. Given these results, the combination of SD-101 + Pembrolizumab is being tested in other tumors.
Another TLR9 agonist is IMO-212 [41]. This is a compound that showed promising results in melanoma in the ILLUMINATE 204 trial in combination with Ipilimumab [42]. However, despite the efficacy in phase 2, the results of phase 3 ILLUMINATE 301 (IMO-212 + ipilimumab vs. ipilimumab) were disappointing [43].

b. **TLR3 agonists**

TLR3 in a receptor located in the endosome capable of recognizing double-stranded RNA [44]. It is mainly expressed on dendritic cells and is responsible for mediating antigen presentation between dendritic cells and lymphocytes. Double-stranded RNA analogs have now been used, as poly I:C-based molecules. BO112, a TLR3 agonist also active against MDA-5 and RIG-I [45], has been tested in different scenarios [46]. The results of phase II testing the efficacy of BO-112 administered intratumorally in combination with pembrolizumab have been encouraging, with 25% response rate in evaluable for response population, which is still better in particular subgroups, such as patients with M1a-N0 disease, who achieved a response rate higher than 70%. Besides, PFS was 16 weeks, which is also a positive result taking into account that all these patients had confirmed progressive disease while on prior immunotherapy [47]. These results need still to be confirmed through randomized trials.

c. **TLR7/8 agonists**

Both TLR7 and TLR8 are receptors located in the endosome [48]. These receptors are capable of recognizing single strands of RNA and triggering the activation of the immune response. Among the most advanced TLR7/8 agonists in development is NKTR-262 [49]. The combination of NKTR-262 administered intratumorally in combination with intravenous BEMPEG is being explored in different tumor types [50]. Although these are preliminary data, it seems that in patients with metastatic melanoma there is some hopeful sign of activity.

d. **STING agonists**

STING pathway activation is triggered by the presence of double-stranded DNA [51]. The activation of this pathway translates into an increase in the response mediated by IFN type I. To date, there are different studies that explore the activation of this pathway using different molecules intratumorally (SYNB1891, CDK-002, BMS-986301, or E7766) [52–56].

4.2 Oncolytic viruses

As previously presented, oncolytic viruses are an important step in the treatment of melanoma. Within the oncolytic viruses administered intratumorally, we have T-VEC (approved by the FDA), PexaVec, and CAVATAK for the treatment of melanoma.

4.3 Other immunity enhancers

Currently, there are different molecules that are being tested and administered with both approaches, intravenous and intratumorally. This is the case with anti-CD40 antibodies. CD40 is a stimulatory signal that enhances the activity of different cells such as macrophages, B and T lymphocytes, as well as antigen-presenting cells. At present, we know encouraging data about the antibodies Selicrelumab [57] (intravenous) and Sotigalimab [58] (intratumoral). Administration of anti-CTLA4 intratumorally has also been investigated with positive signs of efficacy in patients with melanoma [59].

5. Vaccines

Antitumor vaccines have been deeply studied for the past years [60]. Conceptually, it would be based on the administration of selected tumor antigens, as well as other substances that enhance the activation of the immune system (in some cases, dendritic cells, for example, are used per se). This is intended to awaken the acquired response of the host against certain antigens, which would enhance a global response against tumor cells.

Melan A (MART-1), gp100, MAGE, or NY-ESO61 are among the most studied antigens in melanoma [61]. Recently, data from the phase 1/2 trial MM163662 have been presented [62]. In this trial, the role of IO102-IO103 (peptide vaccine composed of IO102 (derived from Indolamine 2,3 dioxygenase (IDO), IO103 (derived from

PDL1), and ISA51 (immunomodulator)) was studied in patients diagnosed with metastatic melanoma. Despite being in the initial phases of research, the data on overall survival, progression-free survival, and response rates are encouraging.

On the other hand, another example of a multi-epitope vaccine was used in trial 18,174 in combination with Pembrolizumab [63]. In this case, the vaccine contained gp100, MelanA/MART-1, two tyrosinase peptides, MAGE-A3 and MAGE-A1,2,3,6 [64]. Despite more modest results, overall survival data in patients who had not been exposed to prior PD1 therapy are promising.

Another different approach was carried out in the phase 2 trial GCO 14–0780 for patients diagnosed with high-risk melanoma and who were treated with complete surgery. This trial studied the efficacy of a poly ICLC-matured dendritic cell vaccine in combination with a peptide vaccine containing NY-ESO and Melan A. This strategy was compared with the administration of Montanide ISA 51 VG and poly ICLC as an adjuvant of the NY-ESO/Melan A vaccine. Results presented at AACR in 2022 showed different degrees of immunization. The effect on relapse-free survival remains to be studied.

On the other hand, there is also a strategy for the development of vaccines based on RNA technology. This is the case of BNT111 [65]. It is a vaccine with RNA encoding for MAGE-A3, NY-ESO1, tyrosinase, and TPTE (putative tyrosine-protein phosphatase). In the phase 1 MERIT study, BNT111 was injected at the lymph node level in patients with metastatic melanoma. The toxicity profile was favorable, so it is currently under development in combination with antiPD1 blockade.

Finally, there is also a vaccination approach against the activity of certain proteins. This is the case of UV1, a vaccine against the catalytic subunit of reverse telomerase (hTERT) [66]. In phase I UV1/hTERT-MM-103 trial, UV1 vaccination was used in combination with Pembrolizumab in patients with metastatic melanoma [67]. The data presented showed interesting results in terms of overall survival and response rate.

6. New therapeutic targets

6.1 Exhausted T cell

Exhausted lymphocytes are defined as lymphocytes with diminished effector functions, as well as compromised cytokine expression [68]. Reversing this state has become a very interesting therapeutic approach since it could be causing both resistance and refractoriness to treatment in some patients. Over the years, certain proteins have been discovered that, when expressed on the surface of lymphocytes, could be contributing to this cellular exhaustion [69]. This is the case with proteins such as LAG3 (lymphocyte activation gene 3) [70] or TIM3 [71](T cell immunoglobulin domain and mucin domain protein 3). Data on Relatlimab (anti-LAG3) in combination with Nivolumab in patients with metastatic melanoma have recently been presented [72]. The positive first-line results of the combination of Relatlimab with Nivolumab versus Nivolumab in patients with metastatic melanoma who had not previously received any line have led to the approval of the combination by the FDA.

There are also drugs that try to block TIM3, although they are less developed. An example of these would be TSR-022 [73] or MBG-453 [74], which could have a promising role in the treatment of melanoma.

6.2 Bispecific antibodies

There are some drugs under development that are capable of binding to two different domains [75]. This is the case of the antiPD1/antiLAG3 [76] or antiPD1/antiTIGIT [77] antibodies. With this approach, the aim is to reduce the "off tumor" side effects while maintaining or even improving efficacy.

6.3 Other therapies

One of the most important discoveries for patients with uveal melanoma has been the development of Tebentafusp [78]. It is composed of a fusion protein containing the human T cell receptor (TCR) specific for the gp100 antigen. At the same time, it is bound to an antibody fragment against CD3. Despite the fact that the drug is currently restricted to those patients with HLA A2:01, it has meant a radical change for a pathology in which there was not an effective alternative [79].

There are currently other trials using TCRs from patients diagnosed with melanoma and who are considered responders to immunotherapy. These TCRs are being tested in patients with different solid tumors (NCT04729543).

7. Conclusions

The treatment of melanoma has dramatically changed over the past few years. The scenario has shifted from barely having drugs available, to having hundreds of trials available for this population. In the future, it is conceivable that just as targeted therapies, it is very likely that we will know the mechanisms of immunoresistance underlying each patient and thus be able to personalize immunotherapy cancer treatments even more.

Author details

Álvaro Sánchez Arráez[1], Sonia Maciá[2*] and Eduardo Castañón[1]

1 Clínica Universidad de Navarra, Spain

2 Highlight Therapeutics, Spain

*Address all correspondence to: smacia@yahoo.com

References

[1] Curti BD, Faries MB. Recent advances in the treatment of melanoma. The New England Journal of Medicine. 2021;**384**(23):2229-2240. DOI: 10.1056/NEJMra2034861

[2] Long GV, Stroyakovskiy D, Gogas H, et al. Combined BRAF and MEK inhibition versus BRAF inhibition alone in melanoma. The New England Journal of Medicine. 2014 Nov 13;**371**(20):1877-1888. DOI: 10.1056/NEJMoa1406037. Epub 2014 Sep 29. PMID: 25265492

[3] Long GV, Flaherty KT, Stroyakovskiy D, et al. Dabrafenib plus trametinib versus dabrafenib monotherapy in patients with metastatic BRAF V600E/K-mutant melanoma: Long-term survival and safety analysis of a phase 3 study. Annals of Oncology. 2017 Jul 1;**28**(7):1631-1639. DOI: 10.1093/annonc/mdx176

[4] Chapman PB, Hauschild A, Robert C, et al. Improved survival with vemurafenib in melanoma with BRAF V600E mutation. The New England Journal of Medicine. 2011 Jun 30;**364**(26):2507-2516. DOI: 10.1056/NEJMoa1103782. Epub 2011 Jun 5. PMID: 21639808; PMCID: PMC3549296

[5] Ascierto PA, McArthur GA, Dréno B, et al. Cobimetinib combined with vemurafenib in advanced BRAF(V600)-mutant melanoma (coBRIM): Updated efficacy results from a randomised, double-blind, phase 3 trial. The Lancet Oncology. 2016 Sep;**17**(9):1248-1260. DOI: 10.1016/S1470-2045(16)30122-X. Epub 2016 Jul 30. PMID: 27480103

[6] Dummer R, Ascierto PA, Gogas HJ, et al. Overall survival in patients with BRAF-mutant melanoma receiving encorafenib plus binimetinib versus vemurafenib or encorafenib (COLUMBUS): A multicentre, open-label, randomised, phase 3 trial. The Lancet Oncology. 2018 Oct;**19**(10):1315-1327. DOI: 10.1016/S1470-2045(18)30497-2. Epub 2018 Sep 12. Erratum in: Lancet Oncology. 2018 Oct;**19**(10):e509. PMID: 30219628

[7] Robert C, Long GV, Brady B, et al. Nivolumab in Previously Untreated Melanoma without *BRAF* Mutation. The New England Journal of Medicine. 2015;**372**(4):320-330. DOI: 10.1056/NEJMoa1412082

[8] Hamid O, Robert C, Daud A, et al. Five-year survival outcomes for patients with advanced melanoma treated with pembrolizumab in KEYNOTE-001. Annals of Oncology. 2019 Apr 1;**30**(4):582-588. DOI: 10.1093/annonc/mdz011. PMID: 30715153; PMCID: PMC6503622

[9] Robert C, Thomas L, Bondarenko I, et al. Ipilimumab plus dacarbazine for previously untreated metastatic melanoma. The New England Journal of Medicine. 2011 Jun 30;**364**(26):2517-2526. DOI: 10.1056/NEJMoa1104621. Epub 2011 Jun 5. PMID: 21639810

[10] Schadendorf D, Hodi FS, Robert C, et al. Pooled Analysis of Long-Term Survival Data From Phase II and Phase III Trials of Ipilimumab in Unresectable or Metastatic Melanoma. Journal of Clinical Oncology. 2015 Jun 10;**33**(17):1889-1894. DOI: 10.1200/JCO.2014.56.2736. Epub 2015 Feb 9. PMID: 25667295; PMCID: PMC5089162

[11] Hodi FS, Chiarion-Sileni V, Gonzalez R, et al. Nivolumab plus ipilimumab or nivolumab alone versus ipilimumab alone in advanced melanoma (CheckMate 067): 4-year outcomes

of a multicentre, randomised, phase 3 trial. The Lancet Oncology. 2018 Nov;**19**(11):1480-1492. DOI: 10.1016/S1470-2045(18)30700-9. Epub 2018 Oct 22

[12] Rosenberg SA. IL-2: The first effective immunotherapy for human cancer. Journal of Immunology. 2014 Jun 15;**192**(12):5451-8. DOI: 10.4049/jimmunol.1490019. PMID: 24907378; PMCID: PMC6293462

[13] Rosenberg SA, Lotze MT, Yang JC, et al. Prospective Randomized Trial of High-Dose Interleukin-2 Alone or in Conjunction With Lymphokine-Activated Killer Cells for the Treatment of Patients With Advanced Cancer, JNCI: Journal of the National Cancer Institute, 21 April 1993;**85**(8):622-632. Available from: https://doi.org/10.1093/jnci/85.8.622

[14] Bentebibel SE, Hurwitz ME, Bernatchez C, et al. A First-in-Human Study and Biomarker Analysis of NKTR-214, a Novel IL2Rβγ-Biased Cytokine, in Patients with Advanced or Metastatic Solid Tumors. Cancer Discovery. 2019 Jun;**9**(6):711-721. DOI: 10.1158/2159-8290.CD-18-1495. Epub 2019 Apr 15. PMID: 30988166

[15] Diab A, Tannir NM, Bentebibel SE, et al. Bempegaldesleukin (NKTR-214) plus nivolumab in patients with advanced solid tumors: Phase I dose-escalation study of safety, efficacy, and immune activation (PIVOT-02). Cancer Discovery. 2020;**10**(8):1158-1173. DOI: 10.1158/2159- 8290.CD-19-1510

[16] Khushalani NI, Diab A, Ascierto PA, et al. Bempegaldesleukin plus nivolumab in untreated, unresectable or metastatic melanoma: Phase III PIVOT IO 001 study design. Future Oncology. 2020 Oct;**16**(28):2165-2175. DOI: 10.2217/fon-2020-0351. Epub 2020 Jul 29. PMID: 32723187

[17] Kaliński P, Hilkens CM, Snijders A, et al. IL-12-deficient dendritic cells, generated in the presence of prostaglandin E2, promote type 2 cytokine production in maturing human naive T helper cells. Journal of immunology, Baltimore, Md. 1997;**159**(1):28-35

[18] Del Vecchio M, Bajetta E, Canova S, et al. Interleukin-12: Biological properties and clinical application. Clinical Cancer Research. 2007 Aug 15;**13**(16):4677-4685. DOI: 10.1158/1078-0432.CCR-07-0776. PMID: 17699845

[19] Daud AI, DeConti RC, Andrews S, et al. Phase I trial of interleukin-12 plasmid electroporation in patients with metastatic melanoma. Journal of Clinical Oncology. 2008 Dec 20;**26**(36):5896-903. DOI: 10.1200/JCO.2007.15.6794. Epub 2008 Nov 24. PMID: 19029422; PMCID: PMC2645111

[20] Daud AI, Algazi AP, Ashworth, et al. Systemic antitumor effect and clinical response in a phase 2 trial of intratumoral electroporation of plasmid interleukin-12 in patients with advanced melanoma. Journal of Clinical Oncology, 32, 9025-9025. DOI: 10.1200/jco.2014.32.15_suppl.9025

[21] Fernandez-Penas P, Carlino M, Tsai K, et al. 383 Durable responses with intratumoral electroporation of plasmid interleukin 12 plus pembrolizumab in patients with advanced melanoma progressing on an anti-PD-1 antibody: Updated data from keynote 695. Journal for Immunotherapy of Cancer. 2021. DOI: 10.1136/jitc-2021-sitc2021.383. (abstract)

[22] Ganesh K, Massagué J. TGF-β Inhibition and Immunotherapy: Checkmate. Immunity. 2018 Apr 17;**48**(4):626-628. DOI: 10.1016/j.

immuni.2018.03.037. PMID: 29669246; PMCID: PMC6347120

[23] Mariathasan S, Turley S, Nickles D. et al. TGFβ attenuates tumour response to PD-L1 blockade by contributing to exclusion of T cells. Nature. 2018;**554**:544-548. Available from: https://doi.org/10.1038/nature25501

[24] Shi M, Chen J, Li K, et al. SHR-1701, a bifunctional fusion protein targeting PD-L1 and TGF-β, for advanced NSCLC with EGFR mutations: Data from a multicenter phase 1 study. Journal of Clinical Oncology. 2021. DOI: 10.1200/jco.2021.39.15_suppl.9055 (abstract)

[25] Kim B-G, Choi SH, Luo G, et al. Vactosertib, a TGF-ß Receptor I Kinase/ ALK5 Inhibitor, Diminishes Tumor Progression and Bone Disease in a Mouse Model of Multiple Myeloma and Overcomes Resistance to Proteasome Inhibitors. Blood. 132. 1918-1918. 10.1182/blood-2018-99-117852

[26] Harrington K, Freeman DJ, Kelly B, et al. Optimizing oncolytic virotherapy in cancer treatment. Nature Reviews Drug Discovery. 2019 Sep;**18**(9):689-706. DOI: 10.1038/s41573-019-0029-0. Epub 2019 Jul 10. PMID: 31292532

[27] Johnson DB, Puzanov I, Kelley MC. Talimogene laherparepvec (T-VEC) for the treatment of advanced melanoma. Immunotherapy. 2015;**7**(6):611-619. DOI: 10.2217/ imt.15.35

[28] Dummer R, Hoeller C, Gruter IP, Michielin O. Combining talimogene laherparepvec with immunotherapies in melanoma and other solid tumors. Cancer Immunology, Immunotherapy. 2017;**66**(6):683-695. DOI: 10.1007/ s00262-017-1967-1

[29] Long G, Dummer R, Johnson D, et al. 429 Long-term analysis of MASTERKEY-265 phase 1b trial of talimogene laherparepvec (T-VEC) plus pembrolizumab in patients with unresectable stage IIIB-IVM1c melanoma. 2020. DOI: 10.1136/jitc-2020-sitc2020.0429. J Immunother Cancer 2020;8(suppl 3)A1-A559

[30] Svane I-M, Santos JM, Cervera-Carrascon V, et al. 1032TiP A phase I, first-in-human, study of TILT-123, a tumor-selective oncolytic adenovirus encoding TNFa and IL-2, in participants with advanced melanoma receiving adoptive T-cell therapy with tumor-infiltrating lymphocytes. Annals of Oncology. 2021;**32**(suppl 5):S864. DOI: 10.1016/j. annonc.2021.08.1416

[31] Beasley GM, Nair SK, Farrow NE, et al. Phase I trial of intratumoral PVSRIPO in patients with unresectable, treatment-refractory melanoma. Journal for Immunotherapy of Cancer. 2021 Apr;**9**(4):e002203. DOI: 10.1136/jitc-2020-002203. PMID: 33875611; PMCID: PMC8057552

[32] Shoushtari AN, Olszanski AJ, Nyakas M, et al. 1083P A pilot study of engineered adenovirus ONCOS-102 in combination with pembrolizumab (pembro) in checkpoint inhibitor refractory advanced or unresectable melanoma. Annals of Oncology. 2021. DOI: 10.1016/j.annonc.2021.08.1468. Poster 1083P

[33] Andtbacka RH, Shafren DR, Grose M, et al. CAVATAK-mediated oncolytic immunotherapy in advanced melanoma patients. 2014. DOI: 10.1158/1538-7445. am2014-2939 (abstract)

[34] Linette GP, Hamid O, Whitman ED, et al. A phase I open-label study of Ad-RTS-hIL-12, an adenoviral vector engineered to express hIL-12 under the control of an oral activator ligand, in

subjects with unresectable stage III/IV melanoma. Journal of Clinical Oncology. 2013. DOI: 10.1200/ jco.2013.31.15_suppl.3022 (abstract)

[35] Champiat S, Tselikas L, Farhane S, Raoult T, Texier M, Lanoy E, et al. Intratumoral Immunotherapy: From Trial Design to Clinical Practice. Clinical Cancer Research. 2021 Feb 1;27(3):665-679. DOI: 10.1158/1078-0432.CCR-20-0473. Epub 2020 Sep 17. PMID: 32943460

[36] Melero I, Castanon E, Alvarez M, et al. Intratumoural administration and tumour tissue targeting of cancer immunotherapies. Nature Reviews Clinical Oncology. 2021 Sep;**18**(9):558-576. DOI: 10.1038/s41571-021-00507-y. Epub 2021 May 18. PMID: 34006998; PMCID: PMC8130796

[37] Hemmi H, Takeuchi O, Kawai T, et al. A Toll-like receptor recognizes bacterial DNA. Nature. 2000 Dec 7;408 (6813):740-755. DOI: 10.1038/35047123. Erratum in: Nature 2001 Feb 1;**409**(6820):646. PMID: 11130078

[38] Kirkwood J, Zakharia Y, Davar D, et al. 950 Final analysis: Phase 1b study investigating intratumoral injection of toll-like receptor 9 agonist vidutolimod ± pembrolizumab in patients with PD-1 blockade–refractory melanoma. Journal for Immunotherapy of Cancer. 2021. DOI: 10.1136/jitc-2021-sitc2021.950 (abstract)

[39] Davar D, Karunamurthy A, Hartman D, et al. 303 Phase II trial of neoadjuvant nivolumab (Nivo) and intra-tumoral (IT) CMP-001 in high-risk resectable melanoma (Neo-C-Nivo): Final results. 2020. DOI: 10.1136/jitc-2020-sitc2020.0303 (abstract). J Immunother Cancer 2020;8(Suppl 3):A1-A559

[40] Amin A, Milhem MM, Long GV, et al. Phase 1b/2, open label, multicenter, study of the combination of SD-101 and pembrolizumab in patients with advanced/metastatic melanoma resistant to anti-PD-1/PD-L1 therapy. Journal of Clinical Oncology. 2019. DOI: 10.1200/ jco.2019.37.15_suppl.9555 (abstract)

[41] Kandimalla ER, Bhagat L, Li Y, et al. Immunomodulatory oligonucleotides containing a cytosine-phosphate-2'-deoxy-7-deazaguanosine motif as potent toll-like receptor 9 agonists. Proceedings of the National Academy of Sciences of the United States of America, 102;**19**:6925-30

[42] Haymaker C, Johnson DH, Murthy R, et al. Tilsotolimod with Ipilimumab Drives Tumor Responses in Anti-PD-1 Refractory Melanoma. Cancer Discovery. 2021 Aug;**11**(8):1996-2013. DOI: 10.1158/2159-8290.CD-20-1546. Epub 2021 Mar 11. PMID: 33707233; PMCID: PMC8544022

[43] Butler MO, Robert C, Negrier S, et al. ILLUMINATE 301: A randomized phase 3 study of tilsotolimod in combination with ipilimumab compared with ipilimumab alone in patients with advanced melanoma following progression on or after anti-PD-1 therapy. 2019;**30**(Suppl 5):v560-v561. ISSN 0923-7534. Available from: https://doi.org/10.1093/annonc/mdz255.061

[44] Alexopoulou L, Holt AC, Medzhitov R, et al. Recognition of double-stranded RNA and activation of NF-kappaB by Toll-like receptor 3. Nature. 2001 Oct 18;**413**(6857):732-738. DOI: 10.1038/35099560. PMID: 11607032

[45] Tormo D, Checińska A, Alonso-Curbelo D, et al. Targeted activation of innate immunity for therapeutic induction of autophagy and apoptosis in melanoma cells. Cancer Cell. 2009 Aug 4;**16**(2):103-14. DOI: 10.1016/j.

ccr.2009.07.004. PMID: 19647221; PMCID: PMC2851205

[46] Aznar MA, Planelles L, Perez-Olivares M, et al. Immunotherapeutic effects of intratumoral nanoplexed poly I:C. Journal for Immunotherapy of Cancer. 2019;7:116. DOI: 10.1186/s40425-019-0568-2

[47] Márquez-Rodas I, de Sanmamed F, Gutiérrez M, Cao MG, et al. Abstract CT233: Phase 2 clinical study to evaluate the efficacy and safety of intratumoral BO-112 in combination with pembrolizumab in patients with advanced melanoma that have progressive disease on anti-PD-1-based therapy. Cancer Research. 2021. DOI: 10.1158/1538-7445.am2021-ct233 (abstract)

[48] Diebold SS, Kaisho T, Hemmi H, Akira S, Reis E, Sousa C. Innate antiviral responses by means of TLR7-mediated recognition of single-stranded RNA. Science. 2004 Mar 5;**303**(5663):1529-1531. DOI: 10.1126/science.1093616. Epub 2004 Feb 19. PMID: 14976261

[49] Diab A, Marcondes M, Tagliaferri MA, et al. REVEAL: A phase I/ II, open-label, multicenter, dose escalation and dose expansion study of NKTR-262 [TLR 7/8 agonist] plus NKTR-214 [CD122-biased agonist] with or without nivolumab (nivo) in patients (pts) with locally advanced or metastatic solid tumor malignancies. Annals of Oncology. 2018. DOI:10.1200/JCO.2019.37.8_SUPPL.26 (abstract)

[50] Diab A, Marcondes M, Kotzin B, et al. Phase Ib: Preliminary clinical activity and immune activation for NKTR-262 [TLR 7/8 agonist] plus NKTR-214 [CD122-biased agonist] in patients (pts) with locally advanced or metastatic solid tumors (REVEAL Phase Ib/II Trial). Journal of Clinical Oncology. 2019. DOI: 10.1200/ jco.2019.37.8_suppl.26 (abstract)

[51] Chen Q, Sun L, Chen ZJ. Regulation and function of the cGAS-STING pathway of cytosolic DNA sensing. Nature Immunology. 2016 Sep 20;**17**(10):1142-1149. DOI: 10.1038/ni.3558. PMID: 27648547

[52] Riese R, Luke J, Lewis K, et al. 500 SYNB1891, a bacterium engineered to produce a STING agonist, demonstrates target engagement in humans following intratumoral injection. J Immunother Cancer 2021;**9**(Suppl 2):A1-A1054 (abstract)

[53] Jang SC, Economides KD, Moniz RJ, et al. ExoSTING, an extracellular vesicle loaded with STING agonists, promotes tumor immune surveillance. Communications Biology. 2021 Apr 22;**4**(1):497. DOI: 10.1038/s42003-021-02004-5. PMID: 33888863; PMCID: PMC8062530

[54] Schieven G, Brown J, Swanson J, et al. P525 Preclinical characterization of BMS-986301, a differentiated STING agonist with robust antitumor activity as monotherapy or in combination with anti-PD-1. Journal for Immunotherapy of Cancer. 2018 (abstract)

[55] Kim DS, Endo A, Fang FG, et al. E7766, a macrocycle-bridged stimulator of interferon genes (STING) agonist with potent pan-genotypic activity. ChemMedChem. 2021 Jun 7;**16**(11):1740-1743. DOI: 10.1002/cmdc.202100068. Epub 2021 Feb 25. PMID: 33522135

[56] Leventhal DS, Sokolovska A, Li N, et al. Immunotherapy with engineered bacteria by targeting the STING pathway for anti-tumor immunity. Nature Communications. 2020 Jun 1;**11**(1):2739. DOI: 10.1038/s41467-020-16602-0. PMID: 32483165; PMCID: PMC7264239

[57] Barlesi F, Lolkema M, Rohrberg KS, et al. 291 Phase Ib study of selicrelumab (CD40 agonist) in combination with atezolizumab (anti-PD-L1) in patients with advanced solid tumors. 2020. DOI: 10.1136/jitc-2020-sitc2020.0291 (abstract)

[58] Weiss S, Sznol M, Shaheen M, et al. 389 Phase II of CD40 agonistic antibody sotigalimab (APX005M) in combination with nivolumab in subjects with metastatic melanoma with confirmed disease progression on anti-PD-1 therapy. Journal for Immunotherapy of Cancer. 2021. DOI: 10.1136/jitc-2021-sitc2021.389 (abstract)

[59] Ray A, Williams MA, Meek SM, et al. A phase I study of intratumoral ipilimumab and interleukin-2 in patients with advanced melanoma. Oncotarget. 2016 Sep 27;7(39):64390-64399. DOI: 10.18632/oncotarget.10453. PMID: 27391442; PMCID: PMC5325451

[60] Saxena M, van der Burg SH, Melief CJM, Bhardwaj N. Therapeutic cancer vaccines. Nature Reviews Cancer. 2021 Jun;**21**(6):360-378. DOI: 10.1038/s41568-021-00346-0. Epub 2021 Apr 27. PMID: 33907315

[61] Maurer DM, Butterfield LH, Vujanovic L. Melanoma vaccines: Clinical status and immune endpoints. Melanoma Research. 2019 Apr;**29**(2):109-118. DOI: 10.1097/CMR.0000000000000535. PMID: 30802228; PMCID: PMC6392068

[62] Kjeldsen JW, Lorentzen CL, Martinenaite E, et al. A phase 1/2 trial of an immune-modulatory vaccine against IDO/PD-L1 in combination with nivolumab in metastatic melanoma. Nature Medicine. 2021 Dec;**27**(12):2212-2223. DOI: 10.1038/s41591-021-01544-x. Epub 2021 Dec 9

[63] Slingluff C, Chianese-Bullock K, Mauldin I, et al. 388 A trial to evaluate the safety, immunogenicity, and clinical activity of a helper peptide vaccine plus PD-1 blockade (Mel64, PATHVACS: PD-1 antibody and T-helper vaccine and correlative studies). J Immunotherapy Cancer, 2021;**9**(2):A1-a1054. DOI: 10.1136/jitc-2021-sitc2021.388

[64] Pavlick AC, Blazquez A, Meseck M, et al. A phase II open labeled, randomized study of poly-ICLC matured dendritic cells for NY-ESO-1 and Mean-A peptide vaccination compared to Montanide, in melanoma patients in complete clinical remission. Journal of Clinical Oncology. 2019. DOI: 10.1200/ jco.2019.37.15_suppl.9538 (abstract)

[65] Sahin U, Oehm P, Derhovanessian E, et al. An RNA vaccine drives immunity in checkpoint-inhibitor-treated melanoma. Nature. 2020 Sep;**585**(7823):107-112. DOI: 10.1038/s41586-020-2537-9. Epub 2020 Jul 29. PMID: 32728218

[66] Ellingsen EB, Mangsbo SM, Hovig E, et al. Telomerase as a Target for Therapeutic Cancer Vaccines and Considerations for Optimizing Their Clinical Potential. Frontiers in Immunology. 2021 Jul 5;**12**:682492. DOI: 10.3389/fimmu.2021.682492. PMID: 34290704; PMCID: PMC8288190

[67] Zakharia Y, O'Day S, Rasch W, Milhem MM. A phase I clinical trial investigating the telomerase vaccine UV1 in combination with pembrolizumab in patients with advanced melanoma. Journal of Clinical Oncology. 2021. DOI: 10.1200/jco.2021.39.15_suppl.2620 (abstract)

[68] Davoodzadeh Gholami M, Kardar GA, Saeedi Y, Heydari S, Garssen J, Falak R. Exhaustion of T lymphocytes in the tumor microenvironment: Significance and effective mechanisms. Cellular Immunology. 2017 Dec;**322**:1-14. DOI:

10.1016/j.cellimm.2017.10.002. Epub 2017 Oct 10. PMID: 29079339

[69] Waldman AD, Fritz JM, Lenardo MJ. A guide to cancer immunotherapy: From T cell basic science to clinical practice. Nature Reviews Immunology. 2020 Nov;20(11):651-668. DOI: 10.1038/s41577-020-0306-5. Epub 2020 May 20. PMID: 32433532; PMCID: PMC7238960

[70] Maruhashi T, Sugiura D, Okazaki IM, Okazaki T. LAG-3: From molecular functions to clinical applications. J Immunother Cancer. 2020 Sep;**8**(2): e001014. DOI: 10.1136/jitc-2020-001014. PMID: 32929051; PMCID: PMC7488795

[71] Wolf Y, Anderson AC, Kuchroo VK. TIM3 comes of age as an inhibitory receptor. Nature Reviews Immunology. 2020 Mar;**20**(3):173-185. DOI: 10.1038/s41577-019-0224-6. Epub 2019 Nov 1. PMID: 31676858; PMCID: PMC7327798

[72] Tawbi HA, Schadendorf D, Lipson EJ, et al. Relatlimab and nivolumab versus nivolumab in untreated advanced melanoma. The New England Journal of Medicine. 2022 Jan 6;**386**(1):24-34. DOI: 10.1056/NEJMoa2109970. PMID: 34986285

[73] Weiss GJ, Luke JJ, Falchook G, et al. A phase 1 study of TSR-022, an anti-TIM-3 monoclonal antibody, in patients (pts) with advanced solid tumors. J Immunother Cancer. 2017 (abstract)

[74] Guru Murthy GS, Atallah E. Targeting TIM-3 as a new strategy in immunotherapy: Focus on sabatolimab. Drugs of the Future. Drugs of the Future. 2021;**46**(11):901. ISSN 0377-8282 e-ISSN 2013-0368. DOI: 10.1358/dof.2021.46.11.3343951

[75] Sheridan C. Bispecific antibodies poised to deliver wave of cancer therapies. Nature Biotechnology. 2021 Mar;**39**(3):251-254. DOI: 10.1038/s41587-021-00850-6. PMID: 33692520

[76] Jiang H, Ni H, Zhang P, et al. PD-L1/LAG-3 bispecific antibody enhances tumor-specific immunity. Oncoimmunology. 2021 Jun 24;**10**(1):1943180. DOI: 10.1080/2162402X.2021.1943180. PMID: 34239776; PMCID: PMC8237984

[77] Bendell JC, Bedard P, Bang Y-J, et al. Abstract CT302: Phase Ia/Ib dose-escalation study of the anti-TIGIT antibody tiragolumab as a single agent and in combination with atezolizumab in patients with advanced solid tumors. Cancer Research. 2020;**80**(16_Suppl): CT302. Available from: https://doi.org/10.1158/1538-7445.AM2020-CT302

[78] Damato BE, Dukes J, Goodall H, Carvajal RD. Tebentafusp: T cell redirection for the treatment of metastatic uveal melanoma. Cancers (Basel). 2019 Jul 11;**11**(7):971. DOI: 10.3390/cancers11070971. PMID: 31336704; PMCID: PMC6679206

[79] Nathan P, Hassel JC, Rutkowski P, et al. Overall survival benefit with tebentafusp in metastatic uveal melanoma. The New England Journal of Medicine. 2021 Sep 23;**385**(13):1196-1206. DOI: 10.1056/NEJMoa2103485. PMID: 34551229